Travel Nurse

Insights

A Window to the World of Travel Nursing

Travel Nurse

Insights

A Window to the World of Travel Nursing

Barry W. Padgett
with Donna E. Padgett, RN, BSN, Traveler

First Edition — First Printing

Buffalo Nickel Publishing LLC

Travel Nurse Insights
A Window to the World of Travel Nursing
Barry W. Padgett with Donna E. Padgett, RN, BSN, Traveler
©2003-2009 Barry W. Padgett

All photographs ©Barry W. Padgett or ©Donna E. Padgett
Cover photo: Autumn Road near Burlington, Vermont
Chapter photos:
  1   Space Needle and Skyline, Seattle
  2   Brooklyn Bridge, New York City
  3   Caesars Palace, Las Vegas
  4   USS Constitution "Old Ironsides", Boston
  5   Saguaro National Park, Tucson, Arizona
  6   Grave Marker, Boothill Graveyard, Tombstone, Arizona
  7   Covered Bridge, Lincoln Gap, Vermont
  8   Golden Gate Bridge, San Francisco
  9   Bald Eagles, Homer, Alaska
  10 Lighthouse at Point Arena, California
  11 Brown Bears Fishing, Brook Falls, Alaska
  12 Welcome Sign, Talkeetna, Alaska
  13 Niagara Falls, New York
  14 Beginning of the Alaska Highway, Dawson Creek, British Columbia
  15 Rodeo Flag Girl, 4th of July, somewhere in America
  16 Fisherman's Memorial, Gloucester, Massachusetts

Opening chapter quotations are by Barry W. Padgett

Published on the 4th of July, 2009
Buffalo Nickel Publishing LLC
P.O. Box 850458
Mobile, Alabama 36685-0458
www.BuffaloNickelPublishing.com

ISBN-10: 0-9821149-0-7
ISBN-13: 978-0-9821149-0-2
Library of Congress Control Number: 2009921886

First Edition
1st printing   February 2009

Printed in the United States of America

Dedicated to all the Grandkids of the World.

(I hope you do a better job running the Planet than we have.)

Caveat

This book is designed to provide general information about the traveling healthcare profession. It is sold with the understanding that neither the author nor the publisher are engaged in rendering accounting, tax, investment, legal, or other professional services. If these or other services are needed, competent professionals should be sought.

The traveling healthcare profession is complicated and varied. To a large extent, each traveler's experience will be unique. Your personal experience may vary radically from ours, and those of your fellow travelers. It is not the purpose of this book to contain all the information available, nor to be exhaustive on any particular topic, but instead to augment, complement, and provide alternative experiences and points of view to other sources of information. This text should be used as a general guide and not as the ultimate or the only information source. It is based on the personal experiences of the author, including discussions with travelers, facilities, agencies, resources of the web, anecdotal information, impressions, and opinions. You are urged to consider all available information and tailor it to your individual circumstances and needs.

Diligent effort has been made to make this publication as complete and accurate as possible. However, there may be mistakes both typographically and in content. This manual contains information on the traveling healthcare profession that is current only to the date of printing or to the referenced date.

Neither the author nor the publisher shall be responsible or liable to any person or entity with respect to loss or damage caused, or alleged to have been caused, directly or indirectly, by the content of this book. If you feel these conditions are inappropriate, please return the book for a full refund.

Contents

Part Three ≈ Ready to Take the Plunge?

Part Four ≈ *Additional Topics*

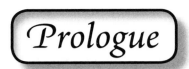

Prologue

S till in her early 50's, she was too young to have these health problems. Headaches were occurring much too often and increasing in severity. In recent years her blood pressure had slowly risen to a level of concern and other related symptoms were beginning to appear. It was becoming apparent: my wife was experiencing job-related stress.

She had been an RN for over twenty years: from ER nurse, to cardiology nurse, to cath lab supervisor and then Director of Cardiology. Her six years as Director were the most challenging. The daily strain of juggling staff and budget, trying to get approval for needed equipment, and the constant meetings and reports to Administration started to show. She felt she needed a change. A chance to step back, catch her breath and start anew.

Something happens when you get a little older. It's difficult to maintain your enthusiasm when you face the same problems day in and day out, year after year. Sure, the exact situations and personnel change but they are really just different versions of the same problems. We had at least two things going for us. Our kids were grown and I was almost eligible to retire from the Federal Government. Maybe we had reached a point in our lives where we could try something else . . . but what?

Two of her employees had left a couple of years earlier to be "travelers". She kept in touch and followed their adventures. They enjoyed traveling: seeing new places, making more money, working where and when they wanted, and enjoying a lot less stress! No longer did they need to deal with hospital politics, internal conflicts, or who was sleeping with whom. They were involved in side issues and personalities only to the extent they wished. They went to work, performed their duties, and focused on good patient care. If the assignment went well they extended. If they wanted to move on they did. As time went by, it all sounded better and better! Could it really be as good as they were saying? Frankly we were skeptical.

I was within a year of being eligible to retire. After 33 years of government service, I needed a change, too! We decided to take the next year to investigate "traveling" to be sure it was right for us. For over thirty years we had lived in the same town working and raising a family. Could we really just pull up roots, throw caution to the wind, and start anew? It was a scary thought! We decided that after the year had passed, if we felt good about it, we would "take the plunge" and begin a whole new life.

We began talking to the agencies our traveler friends recommended. We did a lot of "soul searching" to see if we would like being on the road and away from home for extended periods. As time passed we became more confident about pursuing this new direction.

And when the year was up, we decided to do it! I submitted my retirement papers, my wife gave her notice, her agencies began a serious search for an assignment, and within a month we began the next phase of our life!

We felt confident in our decision to travel but we didn't know much about the industry or the various situations we might encounter. Fortunately our two traveler friends were a great help. They recommended their agencies to us when we were ready to take the plunge. We didn't realize how important that decision is. How lucky we were to get off to a good start!

As we began this new career and talked to fellow travelers, we were surprised how little even some seasoned travelers knew about the profession and about the stipulations of their present assignment. Some barely read their contracts. Were they being paid a reasonable wage? Were reimbursements for living expenses in line for that area of the country? Only after they encountered a problem did they read the contract, and by then it was often too late!

Whether you are a seasoned traveler, a "newbie", or considering a career as a traveler, we believe this book has something to offer. It presents the issues and situations we have encountered either directly or by talking with other travelers, along with healthcare facilities, staffing agencies, and information available on the web. It also contains our impressions and opinions of what we have seen and experienced. It is an ***insight*** into being a traveler. We enjoy traveling and it can be a great experience. But not everything is "wonderful", and traveling is not for everyone. Perhaps by learning from our experiences and those of other travelers, you can avoid mistakes often made.

The book is divided into four parts. The first is an overview of the traveling profession and helps you decide if traveling is right for you. The second discusses the "nitty gritty" topics such as compensation, housing, contracts, and other important items. Together the first two parts help you make an informed decision about traveling. The third part helps prepare you to leave home and survive on the road as a traveler. The fourth contains additional topics of interest.

Traveling is a varied profession. Your experience and the experience of other travelers may differ from ours depending on your choice of agencies, your work ethic, experience, and specialty.

This book is meant to be used! So get out that highlighter, and scribble in the margins and on the note pages. Toss it in the trunk, the back seat of the car, or in the bottom on your suitcase.

During our years of traveling we have taken thousands of photographs and have included a few of our favorites. All photos were taken while on assignment, on nearby trips, or in route to or from assignments. We hope you enjoy them.

In a Nutshell

*H*ere are the major steps involved in traveling:

- ❀ **Decide if traveling is right for you.**

- ❀ **Decide when you wish to begin traveling.**

- ❀ **Choose several agencies to work with.**

- ❀ **Save enough money to cover expenses while you transition to your new career.**

- ❀ **Resign your permanent job, stay PRN, or take a leave of absence to accept a travel assignment.**

- ❀ **Secure your permanent home and pack appropriately.**

- ❀ **Travel to the assignment.**

- ❀ **Move into your new housing.**

- ❀ **Begin work.**

- ❀ **Explore the local area and economy.**

- ❀ **Save money to help you ride through future idle periods.**

- ❀ **During the last few weeks of your assignment, re-evaluate if traveling is right for you.**

- ❀ **Extend your assignment, accept another, take time off, or stop traveling and take a permanent job.**

There you have it! Put this book back on the shelf. No need to read any further!

Well . . . you might want to be aware of just a few of the details.

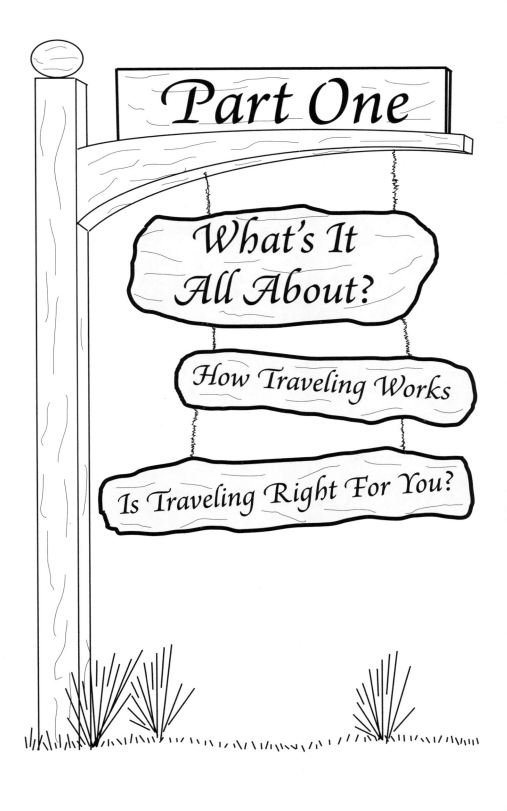

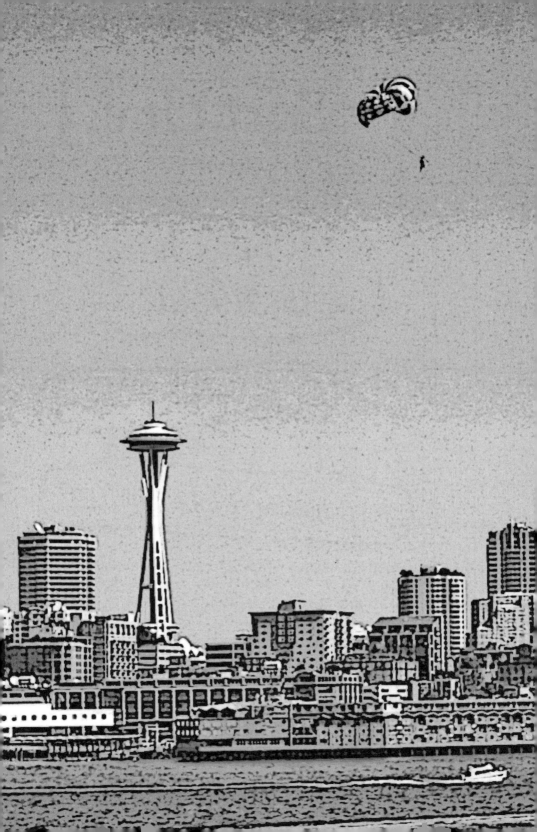

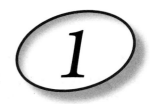

How Traveling Works

I like traveling and seeing this remarkable Nation,
especially when someone else is paying for it.

You have probably heard of "travel nursing" and perhaps even met some travelers. If so, what's your impression: a bunch of free-spirited nurses running around the country, and beyond, working when and where they want? Well . . . that's pretty much it!

Although the profession is best known as "travel nursing" (most travelers are nurses), many other health specialties are included. Even some doctors and dentists travel, filling in as needed. Given the variety of specialties it is probably best to refer to the vocation as the "traveling healthcare profession". Of course, if you're at a cocktail party and tell someone you are a "traveling healthcare professional" be prepared to watch their eyes glaze over as they stumble backwards toward the punch bowl. On the other hand, if you mention you are a "travel nurse", chances are they have some idea of what you are talking about.

Perhaps you have seen those inviting recruitment ads in the medical magazines or on the web. You know, that slick scene of the nurse walking along the beach at sunset carrying her sandals in one hand

and a glass of chardonnay in the other. How about the one with the nurse in the bubble bath with the skyline of New York City in the background? Nice, huh? I'm sure there are places you would like to visit but have never had the chance. Perhaps you would like to see San Francisco, the beaches of Florida, the mountains and deserts of the West, even Alaska or Hawaii. Or maybe you would like to live and work for awhile near a friend or relative that is very special to you. Perhaps you are burned out with your present situation, either professionally or personally, and just need a change.

Now suppose a little birdie landed on your shoulder and whispered, "You can work in the places you have always dreamed of and stay there at least several months. Your housing can be furnished and you can receive extra money to cover your living expenses. You can also receive travel money to and from assignments, and other benefits. In addition to all this you will likely make more per hour than you are making in your present job and enjoy a lot less stress." Sound interesting? It sure did to us! But what's the downside?

Depending on your personality and situation, there may not be one!

Overview of the Industry

The traveling healthcare profession seems to have begun in the late 1970's or the early 1980's. Healthcare facilities in certain regions and some urban areas began having problems maintaining adequate staffing levels. Qualified workers were not entering the field fast enough to keep pace with growing needs, and to replace those leaving.

Staffing agencies began to appear to help fill this need by providing both temporary and permanent healthcare workers. As time has passed the shortage of healthcare professionals has grown. Attempts to control the rising costs of medical care have caused budget cuts and, in some cases, reductions in permanent staff, thus compounding the problem. These staffing shortages have forced those remaining to endure larger patient loads, longer hours, and less time off, adding to the frustration. In addition to retirement, large numbers of professionals have left due to burnout, poor working conditions, and in some cases low pay. Some facilities have increasingly turned to temporary personnel to meet their staffing needs. They can hire and discharge them as the workload varies. However, some facilities find they must continually employ travelers or other temporary workers in order to meet their needs. So the three major components of the traveling healthcare industry are:

The Facility needing staff

The Staffing Agency providing temporary workers

The Traveler willing to accept short term assignments

Traveling vs. Per Diem

Temporary employees may be available through local per diem registries maintained by the facilities or staffing agencies. These workers live within commuting distance and work as needed, sometimes on short notice. Some may have an agreement or contract to work certain days and certain hours per week. They almost always have several things in common: they work only part-time, make more per hour than their counterparts, live close enough to commute, and have few if any benefits.

On the other hand, the traveler is a ***full time*** temporary worker. They sign a contract to work for a specific period; normally 13 weeks (1/4 of a year). Most often they work too far from their home to commute, and must relocate. They are often placed by a staffing agency but may also work directly for the facility, or work as an independent contractor finding their own assignment.

The staffing agency provides housing, living expenses, benefits, and pays the traveler, recouping its cost and making a profit from the facility. The traveler can often qualify for tax advantages based on the fact they are temporarily employed away from their permanent home.

The Facility's View

Not every facility needs temporary employees, but many do. Each facility is responsible for hiring qualified workers to provide the best healthcare possible. They try to maintain staffing levels, contend with changing budget constraints, and referee problems among staff, other units, and with the doctors. As time has passed, many facilities have seen their staff reduced by normal attrition or as part of a budget cutting process. When they get the approval to hire, they would prefer to fill new positions with permanent workers that live in the area: those that have local ties and plan to stay. But given the national nursing shortage, it may be difficult to find enough qualified local permanent workers. Occasionally, it would help to hire temporary workers to fill in for permanent staff that are injured or ill for prolonged periods, or out for such things as vacation, maternity, or family leave.

One solution is to simply live with the shortage. That is, have the permanent employees take more patients per shift, work more overtime, take more call, etc. While this may help in the short run, it can take a toll on the effectiveness and morale of the staff.

Another solution is to work with agencies or registries to hire local per diem workers. This allows the facility to employ workers on a short term basis, perhaps even daily. It also assumes that a large enough pool of such workers exists in the area.

Yet another solution is to contract with one or more staffing agencies to provide travelers. These full-time qualified and experienced workers can augment the permanent staff. The facility can adjust the staffing level by increasing or decreasing the number of travelers as their needs change.

Those facilities needing travelers sometimes prefer to deal with only one agency. This makes things easier for them. Of course, this assumes the agency can always provide competent travelers at a reasonable price. Other facilities deal with multiple agencies and let them compete to fill openings, and will establish new contracts with agencies if they think they can get a better deal or can fill their needs more quickly. Still others have their own in-house staffing agency. A few facilities hire a vendor manager. This is usually an independent staffing agency that acts as the facility's agent in dealing with other agencies providing travelers. They screen the agencies and only establish contracts with those that agree to the facility's terms.

Even after the facility hires a traveler there are still unanswered questions. Sure, the traveler looks good on paper and the interview went well, but are they really as qualified as they appear? Will their personality mesh well with the permanent staff? And if things go well, will they stay for awhile or leave after their initial contract ends? The facility will then have to start from scratch and take a chance on yet another traveler! There is some good news for the facility in all of this. It is much easier to get rid of a problem traveler than it is to terminate a permanent staff member.

The Role of the Staffing Agency

The staffing agency acts as the intermediary between the health-care facility and the traveler. It is responsible for providing qualified candidates to the facility. This relieves the facility of much of the pre-employment screening that occurs when they hire permanent employees. The screening by the agency helps assure the facility that the traveler is at least minimally qualified to fill the need.

Once you have chosen one or more agencies to work with (more about this later), submit your application, references, skills checklist and other information to them. Based on this information, the agency will create a "profile" to submit to facilities. This is a summary of your education, experience, and credentials. Think of it as a form of resume. They attempt to match your abilities with the current needs of their facilities. When your agency has an assignment for you, with your permission, they will "present" you to the facility by sending them your profile.

If the facility likes what they see, they call your agency and arrange for a telephone interview with you. This is your chance to learn specifics about the assignment to be sure it is right for you. If this goes well and the facility wants you to work with them, your agency sends you a contract for the assignment. After you agree to the terms and sign your contract, the agency makes all necessary travel and housing arrangements depending on your circumstances (more about this later). As mentioned, the contract period is usually for 13 weeks, although shorter or longer assignments are possible.

The agency has a separate contract with the facility. It defines the hourly "bill rate" and other stipulations between the two. The bill rate is the amount paid the agency for each working hour of the normal work week and depending on the specialty may be in the range of $55-$78 (and more) per hour. There are also stipulations regarding the overtime rate, shift differentials, call back, etc. This rate may seem rather high especially when you consider how much you are making per hour! Keep in mind that from this the agency makes its profit, pays your wage, provides housing, and pays items such as a daily living expense and travel costs. Also, based on its income from all travelers under contract, the agency provides group benefits such as medical and dental coverage, life insurance, 401(k) services, malpractice insurance, etc. We'll talk more about how the bill rate "pie" is allocated in Chapter 11.

How does an agency establish a contract with a facility? They have to convince them they can provide qualified travelers at an acceptable price. The agency "markets" their travelers by way of "blind" profiles. This involves informing the facility of their travelers, not by name, but by experience, education, and credentials. This gives the facility at least some confidence the agency has the ability to fill the needs as they arise.

Your Role as a Traveler

The facility is counting on your experience and knowledge to provide help for the permanent staff. They expect you to be fully proficient with only minimal orientation and training.

The successful traveler adopts a whole new mind set. No longer are you tied to one job in one location. You are a "freelancer" and accept assignments of your choosing. Unlike your old permanent job, each assignment stands alone. Once your contract is fulfilled you are under no further obligation to the facility or the agency. At the end of your contract you have several options. You can agree to extend your contract if the facility still wants and needs you, or you can accept another assignment with that same agency (or with another), accept a permanent position somewhere, take some time off, whatever.

You may think you work for the agency, and I suppose in a legal sense you do. After all, you sign a contract to accept an assignment through them. However, the agency may owe its very existence to the hard work of you and others under contract. Without that income they could be out of business. So in a sense they work for you. You are driving the train! I like to think of it as a team effort: the agency finds the opening and handles many of the details. The traveler generates income for themselves and the agency.

A Win-Win-Win Situation

In the business world they often speak of the need to create "win-win" situations. Both parties to a deal feel it is beneficial to them. Traveling may actually be a "win-win-win" situation. If handled correctly, the facility wins, your agency wins, and you win.

The facility wins because they can augment their permanent staff with temporary personnel. This allows them to adjust their staff to changes in case load and budget. They do not have to keep a large number of permanent staff onboard to satisfy the worst case scenario. They contract only for the period needed; extending or canceling contracts as required. They do not directly pay the benefits they pay their permanent staff. Your agency provides that via your hourly wage and other payment items.

Your agency wins because they can make a living providing qualified health professionals to facilities that need them.

And you win because you get to travel to places you have always wanted to see, have someone else pay for it, have them make all (or most) of the arrangements, and most likely make more money than you made in your old job.

How Openings Are Filled

In a "perfect world" here's how openings would be filled. The facility calls their staffing agency under contract and gives them a list of their new needs. The agency happens to have the exact number of travelers with the correct specialty (who are also just finishing up their current assignment) to fill the needs. The travelers are presented, the facility interviews them, finds them acceptable, and contracts are issued to the travelers. Everyone reports to work on time, has their license, and just absolutely loves their housing. End of story, right?

This scenario may play out occasionally, but I suspect it's not the norm. At last count there were well over 200 agencies in the U.S. placing travelers. Competition is fierce. Even if an agency has an exclusive contract with a facility, they may not have travelers available in the right specialty when the facility needs them. The agency may convince the facility that they can meet their needs shortly. Perhaps they have travelers that will be available soon. If this is not acceptable, the facility may choose to contact other agencies to see if they can meet the needs. Agencies may also subcontract through other agencies to provide travelers in a timely manner.

It gets more complicated when the facility has contracts with more than one agency. They may give some lead time to the agency that usually provides travelers at a lower cost. If that agency can't fill the need, the other agencies are given a chance. If no agency under contract can fill the need, the facility can contact still other agencies. All the while the facility is trying to hire permanent staff to avoid the use of travelers.

If an outside agency hears the details of an opening and has a qualified traveler available, they can contact the facility, present the traveler, and possibly fill the opening. Also, if a traveler hears of an opening they can ask their agency to try to get them there. Their agency can then contact the facility, present the traveler, and attempt to fill the opening. This cut-throat operation by some has led agencies to be rather secretive about their openings. Good agencies attempting to pay their travelers well usually do not advertise too many details of their openings for fear of being undercut by a competitor. They prefer serious candidates contact them directly to get the full details.

During the Civil War, Southern General Nathan B. Forrest was asked how he had been so successful in battle. He purportedly said, "Git thar first with the most". Filling needs is sometimes like that. They can remain open for extended periods while several agencies scramble to fill them. Agencies and the facility will advertise the openings and offer incentives in an attempt to find qualified candidates. In this free-for-all environment whoever "gits thar first" with qualified candidates fills the openings.

> *Insight*
>
> *Openings can also be filled by word of mouth. The facility may ask their current travelers to recommend someone they know. The travelers can call those they have worked with to see if any are interested. If this results in a placement (especially if an agency establishes a new contract with the facility) a referral bonus should be given to the traveler who initiated the process.*

Here are some additional factors that affect the filling and availability of openings:

Variations in pay. If you are a seasoned traveler you have experienced this. Not every location pays the same for the same specialty. While there are exceptions in every area, places in the South tend to pay a little less. I suspect it relates to the lower cost of living and perhaps the milder winter climate. Certain areas of Florida may pay less, probably because they feel they can entice travelers to their beaches or other attractions. Areas where the nursing shortage has hit the hardest often pay more to entice qualified candidates.

A few states use hospital associations to attempt to moderate costs. Member facilities are expected to adhere to the established guidelines. If you want to go there, you (and your agency) play by their rules. Some travelers avoid these areas, seeking opportunities elsewhere. Vendor managers and sole agency contracts are also used to help gain efficiency.

Desirability of the area. Desirability is in the eye of the beholder. Some find the inner city or the more remote regions of the country less desirable. Such areas may have to pay more to attract travelers. Other areas may be "seasonally undesirable". The Northeast is a great area, but winters can be harsh. Summer in portions of the desert Southwest can be uncomfortable to some. Resort areas may pay less because travelers often want to go there regardless of the lower pay.

The reputation of the facility. Many facilities have an excellent reputation in dealing with travelers and can often draw the most qualified candidates. Conversely, some facilities have a poor reputation for dealing with travelers. Even some individual units within otherwise good facilities suffer from this. As word spreads they may have difficulty filling needs.

Nursing schools in the area. Some areas of the country have a sufficient pool of graduating healthcare workers to satisfy the local need. Such areas will have few opportunities for travelers and even local per diem workers.

Economic conditions. Periodically the U.S. economy experiences a downturn. Charitable contributions to facilities from individuals and endowments may be scaled back. Patients having serious illness or injury will almost certainly seek treatment. But they may postpone routine tests, examinations, and elective procedures in order to save money, further reducing the facility's income. Travelers may find it harder to land a desirable assignment during tough economic times.

It is difficult for a facility to hire travelers if the permanent staff jobs are in jeopardy.

National nursing shortage. Regardless of good pay or desirable locations there are, arguably, not enough healthcare professionals to cover all the needs.

Areas of Expertise Needed

Almost any area related to healthcare has a need for travelers. Here are some of the specialties:

- Cardiovascular Intensive Care (CVICU)
- Cardiovascular Lab
- Dentists
- Echo Tech
- Emergency Department (ED)
- Home Healthcare
- Hospice
- Intensive Care Unit (ICU)
- Interventional Radiology (IR)
- Labor and Delivery (L&D)
- Medical Doctors
- Medical/Surgical (MedSurg)
- Medical Technologist
- Neonatal Intensive Care Unit (NICU)
- Nuclear Medical Tech
- Operating Room (OR)
- Pediatrics
- Pharmacist
- Physical Therapist (PT)
- Post Anesthesia Care Unit (PACU)
- Radiology
- Rehabilitation Therapist
- Respiratory Therapist
- Speech Pathologist (SLP)
- Telemetry

And several degree/certification programs are represented:

* Bachelor of Science in Nursing (BSN)
* Cardiovascular Tech (CVT)
* Certified Nurse Anesthetist (CRNA)
* Chemotherapy certification
* Licensed Practical Nurse (LPN)
* Licensed Vocational Nurse (LVN)
* Nurse Practitioner (NP)
* Radiology Tech (AART)
* Registered Cardiovascular Interventional Specialist (RCIS)
* Registered Nurse (RN)
* Registered Nurse First Assistant (RNFA)

Seasonal Assignments

Certain areas of the country experience an increase in population during portions of the year. Florida, Arizona, and New Mexico come to mind because of their moderate winter climate. Other western states, especially Colorado, Utah, and parts of California experience an active winter ski season. During these periods, seasonal assignments may be available as well as regular travel assignments. Seasonal assignments are usually handled directly through the facilities. They post jobs, interview, and sign contracts directly with travelers and other temporary employees. They generally offer a good hourly wage but fewer benefits. Some offer housing or a housing stipend but may offer only limited per diem, travel, or other tax-free reimbursements. But again you may make more per hour than with a traditional agency.

If you wish to accept a seasonal assignment directly through the facility, be sure you understand all the details, especially what costs you will have to bear. Also, be sure to investigate the housing location and availability.

Working as an Independent Contractor

I suspect most travelers are like us. We want our agencies to find good assignments, provide benefits, housing (or a stipend), pay us on time, withhold taxes, etc. In exchange, we are happy to give them their profit margin to avoid this hassle.

However you may ask, "Why go through an agency at all? Why not contract directly with the facility and pocket the full bill rate?" Some travelers choose this option and become Independent Contractors (IC), acting in their own behalf. There is more money to be made as an IC if you are willing to assume this added responsibility.

In its truest form, the IC is not only the traveler but fulfills the duties of the agency. They locate their jobs and handle all the negotiating and contracting details with the facility. They bill the facility for their services, pay estimated taxes, and provide their own benefits such as housing, healthcare, life insurance, professional insurance, retirement account, etc. The IC usually creates a legal business entity such as a "C", "S", "LLC" corporation or a sole proprietorship. While this does not require a formal business office, they may need an office capability including a business phone and a printer/fax. Some IC's print brochures, business cards, and specialized forms for business use.

Another form of independent contractor exists. An agency finds the opening and places the IC. The agency handles only the payment between the facility and the IC. This allows a more timely flow of money to the IC instead of having to wait as long as 45 days to receive payment directly from the facility. The IC is still responsible for everything else previously mentioned. The agency charges a small administration fee, perhaps $5.00 per hour, for this service and the IC receives the remainder of the bill rate.

Well, you can see this can be quite involved, and more than many travelers want to do. If you wish to pursue this form of traveling, you can search the web using a search string such as "independent nursing contractor". Several web sites are available to provide detailed information and Delphi Forums has a discussion group titled "Independent Nurses".

Notes

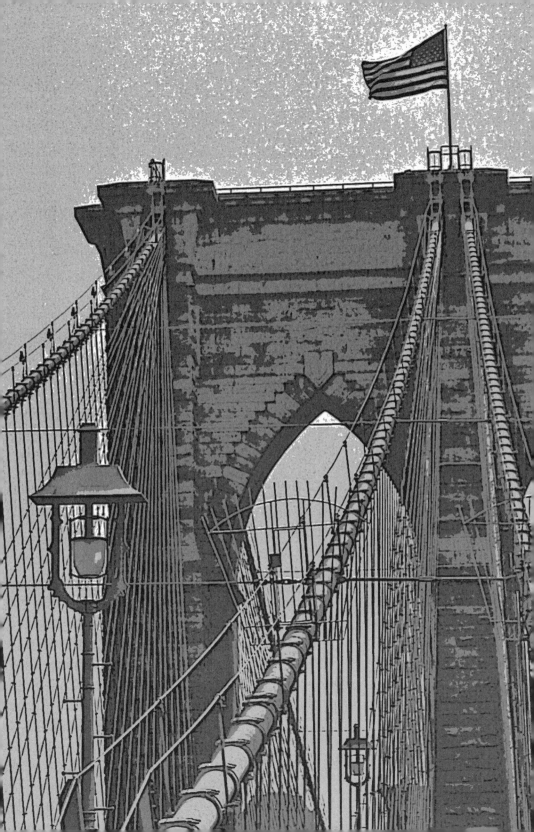

2

Is Traveling Right For You?

*Moving every few months keeps Life interesting.
By the time I figure out what time zone I'm in it's time
to pack up again.*

*D*o you think you might want to try traveling? The decision is important and needs careful consideration. After all you will be leaving your comfort zone: your permanent home, your personal ties, and your permanent job. Take your time. You can tough it out at your old job long enough to be sure it is right for you. We spent one year investigating traveling before we began.

An Important Decision

Changing jobs is always stressful, even if you are looking forward to the future. You should discuss it with your family, close friends, and trusted coworkers. If possible, talk to travelers directly to see how they like it and what issues may apply to you. Tune into web discussion forums related to traveling to read about some of the current issues and concerns (more about this later). Of course, if you try it and find it is not what you want, you can almost certainly accept a permanent staff position. And the way things are going with the nursing shortage, you may be able to return to the exact same job you left!

Many travelers remain PRN at their old job, accept one or more travel assignments, then return home to work locally for extended periods before traveling again.

Traveling will be a significant change in your life style. You will encounter new challenges, constantly meet new people, learn to handle different equipment, and learn different procedures. Local customs and regional slang can sometimes be a challenge. But this is also part of the fun and excitement.

As a permanent staffer you have a certain routine to your life. You go to the same place each workday, see the same coworkers, have the same friends, and return home after work to your familiar surroundings. In other words you have "predictability" in your life. On the road, much of that changes. Each assignment will present a unique situation to which you must adapt. One of the first things our recruiter told us was to be flexible. How true this is! But again, this is part of the adventure.

Characteristics of a Good Traveler

You must be qualified. Are you qualified to be a traveler? Most agencies require at least one year of clinical experience in your specialty prior to accepting an assignment. More experience may be required if you are in a highly specialized or technical area. Of course, the more experience the better. You will also need the appropriate certifications and, if required, a license to practice in that state. Keep in mind when facilities hire travelers they need help. They generally don't have the time or resources for on-the-job training. Travelers need to be fully qualified to perform the duties with minimal training and orientation. Occasionally, you may find a facility so desperate for help they are willing to train a traveler. But this is not the norm.

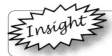

Travelers are sometimes hired to train new permanent staff members.

Work well with others. You need to fit in well with your fellow workers. Remember, you are there to fill in and augment the permanent staff. You are not there to change the world. If you have suggestions for improvements, do so tactfully and always work through the chain of command. Take your time getting to know your coworkers. Do your best to fit into their professional and social setting. I suggest avoiding in depth discussions regarding politics or religion. They can alienate and may cause hard feelings.

Be flexible. Each facility, and indeed every work area, may have procedures and scheduling options you have not encountered. Before suggesting changes learn their procedures and try to fit in as best you can. Even if some procedures and policies do not seem to make sense at first, there may be valid reasons for them.

Ignore the local politics. Each area has its own office politics. Be friendly to all and avoid taking sides in turf issues. The problems you encounter when you arrive will be there long after you take another assignment!

Be confident. You need to be confident: both personally and professionally. You will experience new situations and personalities. When you first arrive, almost everyone will be aware you are probably making more money than they are. They should be happy to have the additional help, but there can be some resentment. Your confidence and skill will help you gain acceptance.

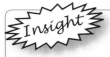

And please don't confuse confidence with arrogance. You need the former. No one wants to put up with the latter!

Advantages of Traveling

Earn more money. Some use traveling as a way to increase their income. Who wouldn't like that? Some need help with their monthly bills, others want to pay off certain debts, or save for a special purpose such as the down payment for a house or college costs for a child or grandchild.

Depending on your specialty you will most likely earn more money per hour traveling than in your permanent job. In addition, you can receive extra pay for living expenses while on the road. Depending on your tax status these allowances may be tax-free. This can add substantially to your income without increasing your tax burden.

So how much more can you earn as a traveler? Think about how much you bring home now as a permanent staffer. Even if you made the exact same hourly wage, tax-free reimbursements can add 20% to 30% more to your bottom line. Now that's what I call a raise!

Choose your time off. Would you like to be off every Christmas? How about every Thanksgiving? You can! By planning the start and end dates of your contracts, using contract extensions, and by specifying individual dates off during the contract period, you can be off almost literally whenever you want.

Work less per year. Some use the higher income to allow them to work less per year. If you can manage your debt and increase your savings enough, you may reach a point where you can be off for extended periods throughout the year.

Travel. Many accept assignments for the adventure of going to new and exciting places . . . and letting someone else pay for it!

Take mini-vacations. Even while on assignment, short excursions on a three or four day weekend can enhance your traveling experience. Some take extra time getting to and from assignments; stopping along the way to see the sights.

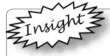 *While driving home from Alaska, we visited three national parks in Canada and five in the U.S. without going too far out of the way.*

Escape. Traveling can help some escape their present situation, either professional or personal. Perhaps you are burned out in your local setting and just need a change of pace. Getting away can allow you to start anew, and rekindle your positive attitude.

Meet new people. It is always exciting to meet new and interesting people. Many will have a varied experience from yours and have different, interesting points of view. Some use traveling as a way to look for their lifelong partner.

Search for a permanent job. You can investigate areas of the country you may wish to reside. Working for several months in a locality can give you the real flavor for both the area and the local employment opportunities.

Expand your knowledge. Traveling gives you the opportunity to see how situations are handled in different areas of the country. You can often learn new techniques, use different equipment, and sometimes expand your knowledge and experience into other specialties.

Visit a relative or friend. You may want to spend an extended period with a family member or friend living away from you. Perhaps they need special care, or you want to be near during a certain point in their life, such as for that of a young grandchild.

Disadvantages of Traveling

Frankly, traveling is not for everyone. Here are some issues to consider:

You are a temporary worker. Unlike your permanent job, you are now a temporary contract worker. You are obligated to that facility and agency only for the life of the existing contract. And of course, this also means they are only obligated to you for that same period. While this gives you freedom to pick your assignments and your times off, there is almost always a contract clause stating your assignment can be terminated without cause at any time. No fuss . . . no muss. The facility just picks up the phone, calls your agency and you are on the next bus out of there! While this possibility may be somewhat disturbing, most facilities go out of their way to honor their contracts even if their needs change. After all, many count on travelers to fill their needs. A reputation for treating travelers poorly can hurt their future relationships with travelers and staffing agencies.

Occasionally needs of the facility change suddenly dictating reduced staffing levels. If this happens and you are terminated early, your agency should do their best to find you another job as soon as possible.

> *Insight* — *If a traveler is discharged prior to completion of the contract, it is often due to a personality conflict, whether justified or not. Given the nursing shortage, if you are experienced, qualified, and get along well with others, the chance of being terminated early is just about nil.*

You will be away from home for extended periods. Traveling is fun and exciting. But it's also tiring in the sense of being away from home, family, and close friends. Sure, you meet new people and make friends on the road. This helps, but honestly it's not the same. As Dorothy in "The Wizard of Oz" discovered, there really is no place like home.

There is a certain sense of security associated with having a permanent job and living in your own home with "your stuff" around you. Some are not as adventurous as others and do not adapt well to changing situations. Moving to a new job in a different part of the country every few months can be too stressful for some.

Lack of paid time off. One of the benefits of working as a full time permanent staffer is the chance to accumulate paid time off. This bank of hours allows you to be off periodically and still receive your full-time pay.

As a traveler you will have little or no paid time off. Some agencies will allow up to three sick days per 13 week assignment and perhaps a week's pay if you work a year or more with them. But travelers tend to change agencies fairly often and may take off for extended periods throughout the year. As such you may seldom qualify for much paid time off. Your savings will have to sustain you during your idle periods.

Maintaining your personal relationships. Being separated for long periods is not conducive to your relationship with your spouse, your children, and others.

Those with family members requiring at least periodic care. It is difficult to provide care and support to those you love while away for extended periods.

Those with local business ties. If you have responsibilities to a family business or other endeavor in your local area, traveling may be difficult. It may be too much of a hardship to be away for long periods.

Examine Your Marketability

As with any job, the more valuable you are, the better your chances of getting the location you want and the pay you feel you deserve. Here are some things that can strengthen your negotiating position and marketability.

Your specialty. While almost any field in the healthcare industry uses travelers, some specialties pay more and are in more demand than others. The agencies can give you guidance as to what availability and range of hourly wage you should expect. You may experience extended periods of unemployment as a traveler if your specialty or credentials for that specialty are not in high demand.

Extent of experience. As you would expect, the more experience you have in your field the more valuable you become. All things being equal, you would expect the person with the most related experience to have the best chance of being chosen for the assignment.

Good evaluations and professional recommendations. Agencies and facilities are looking for people that consistently do a good job and can fit in well. A history of good evaluations will increase your marketability. Several letters of recommendation from doctors you have worked with will also help.

License, certifications, and activities. Be sure you have the required license and certifications, and that they are current. Membership in organizations related to your field will indicate you are truly serious about your profession.

Flexibility. Are you willing to accept assignments in a wide range of locations? Are you willing to float or cross train in other areas? The more flexibility you have the more opportunities will be available.

Versatility. Are you already qualified and willing to work in multiple specialties? This can add marketability and help land that special assignment.

Accepting Assignments Close To Home

Some of the disadvantages of traveling can be eased by accepting assignments close to home. This allows you to return frequently and reduces the feeling of separation. You may be able to arrange longer shifts, say 10 or 12 hours to take advantage of three or four day weekends.

Insight *Check with your tax advisor to be sure you understand any tax implications of working close to home. Depending on how close your assignment is to your permanent home, some of your income may not qualify for the tax-free status usually associated with traveling. We discuss this further in Chapter 6 on taxes.*

Traveling With Others

For many, being on the road can get lonely. Having a friend, family member, or a pet traveling with you can make the journey easier. Here are some of the travel combinations:

With your spouse or significant other. Some travelers have a spouse or significant other that is free to travel with them. Perhaps they are also a traveler, retired, or in a line of work that is not hindered by traveling.

With children. Raising children is a challenge under the best of conditions. Moving them potentially several times a year presents a special challenge. While this might work when the children are preschool age, when they get older it could be difficult. Some travelers, with spouses or significant others, home school their children while on assignment. This takes a special parent-child relationship to make it work. I suspect many would find it difficult to successfully home school while on the road. However, if you wish to pursue home school-ing, enter it as a search string into your browser. There are many web sites and support groups available. Be aware that the requirements for testing and reporting vary among the different States.

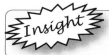 *Frankly, if you have school age children living with you, I recommend you think twice about traveling.*

With another healthcare worker. Traveling with another health-care worker presents some interesting possibilities. Whether it is a spouse, significant other, a friend, or relative, you can share costs and pocket more money. Keep in mind it will require more effort by an agency to place both of you at the same facility, or in the general area, for the same duration.

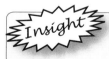 *This situation may present problems if for some reason one has to leave the assignment before the other, espe-cially if you are married or have a significant other.*

With pets. Here's a question for all you seasoned travelers that take your pets with you and have your agency provide housing. When you first considered traveling, what did your recruiter tell you about trav-eling with pets? It was probably something like, "Oh, yes! Pets are no problem. It can make the travel experience so much more enjoyable to bring them along!" Sounded good, didn't it?

And then when it came to finding affordable housing (especially in or near a large city) what did they say? You probably heard something like, "Well, you know, your pet is an issue. It's difficult to find good housing reasonably close to work that also accepts pets."

The point is if you enjoy a pet and wish it as a companion, you may have to accept somewhat of a step-down in housing quality and may have to endure a longer commute to work. It is not such a problem in smaller, rural areas of the country, but in larger, more crowded areas, it can be a housing drawback to travel with a pet.

There can also be extra housing costs associated with pets. Pet deposits and other fees are often charged. Some are not refundable. Be aware up front if there are any special pet fees, and if your agency will cover them. This can be a contract negotiation point with your agency. We'll talk about issues with pets again in Chapter 3 on housing.

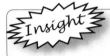 *Should all this discourage you from traveling with your pet? By no means! We traveled with two dogs and chose assignments accordingly.*

Internet Resources

It's difficult to imagine surviving in this day and age without a computer connected to the internet. This is especially true if you are a traveler. Between e-mail, online banking, and finding your favorite stores while on assignment, the web is often your connection to the world.

Bookmarks and search strings are invaluable. Once you find a great resource, bookmark it for future reference. I would also suggest using search strings often. For instance, if you are trying to find rental car companies enter "rental cars" as a search string. Web sites often change their home page address, and new, related web sites are always appearing. Using search strings will bring up the latest site addresses for you to bookmark and also show related sites you may not have otherwise considered. I suggest using a couple of search engines. They sometimes produce different results.

The internet provides a wealth of information about the various issues of the traveling healthcare industry. Web sites include tips on taxes, dealing with facilities and agencies, traveling in RV's, working in foreign countries, the Nurse Licensure Compact, and many other topics. You can enter search strings such as "travel nurse", "travel nursing", "travel nurse companies", "travel nurse jobs", etc., to help find the latest sites. There are also discussion forums on the web dealing with all aspects of life. You can focus on those dealing with traveling by entering a search string such as "travel nurse forums" or perhaps "nursing forums" to help locate them. I suggest visiting at least www.pantravelers.org, www.travelnursetoolbox.com, www.nursetraveler.org, and www.highwayhypodermics.com. All have good information on traveling. Travel Nurse Toolbox also has a comprehensive list of agencies and Highway Hypodermics compares agencies that have responded to a survey.

The Delphi discussion forums (www.delphiforums.com) are also noteworthy. While they deal with many of life's topics, several are specific to the traveling healthcare profession. Members read and post information and opinions on a full range of issues. Recruiters can also post jobs and otherwise participate in the exchange. Basic membership is free and will allow you to read and post messages. You can also search back several months for the most recent posts on any subject. To go back further you will need to increase your membership level and pay a little per month. Here are a few Delphi forums you may wish to visit:

- Travel Nurses & Therapists-No Recruiting (also called TNT)
- TNT Recruiting Board – sister board of the above
- ER Nurses
- Independent Nurses
- Laboratory Professionals
- OB Nurses Forum
- Operating Room Travelers
- Travel Nurse Housing
- Travel Psych Nurses

- ❋ Nurses on Wheels
- ❋ Traveling Radiology Techs

To access these or other Delphi forums, enter the name of the forum in the upper left search box of the Delphi Forums home page. Then bookmark the forum for easier access next time.

> **Insight** *Forums are a great source of information. Unfortunately, some travelers have experienced problems and are not completely unbiased when posting opinions of agencies and recruiters. And of course the one telling the story is **never** at fault! It is difficult for recruiters to defend themselves without looking petty and unprofessional. However, if you read several posts over time that basically say the same thing, you can have some confidence in their opinions. Just take it all with a grain of salt.*

By using this book, other publications, and the vast resources of the internet, you should be able to decide if traveling is right for you.

The next section of the book, Part Two, discusses the "nitty gritty" issues important to every traveler. We'll start right after . . .

A Quick Word About Licensing

If you decide to travel and are required to have a license to practice, you may wish to apply ahead of time to at least those states you are sure you want to visit. In this age of increased security, licensing can take longer than you might expect. Fingerprinting and background checks are the norm. By applying to those states, even before you leave your permanent job, you will have a head start toward getting that special assignment when it is offered. The Nurse Licensure Compact can ease the licensing process, if you are able to take advantage of it. See Chapter 9 for more details on licensing and the Compact. Agencies will often reimburse you for the licensing costs required for your assignment.

Notes

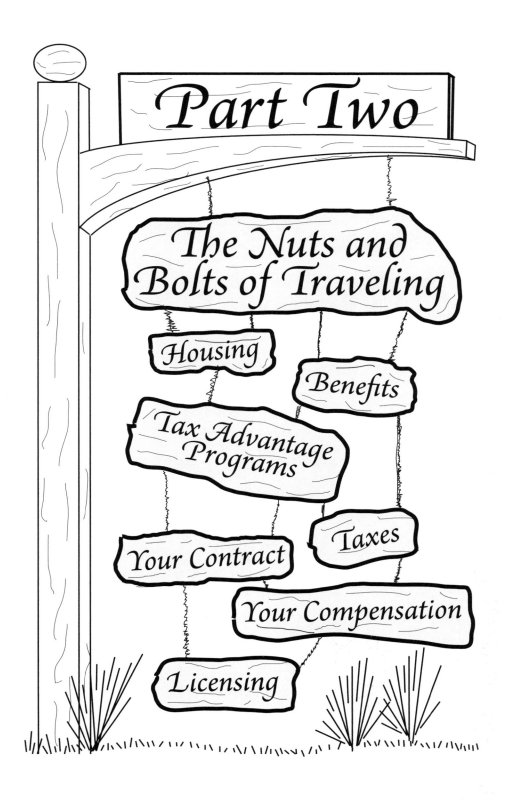

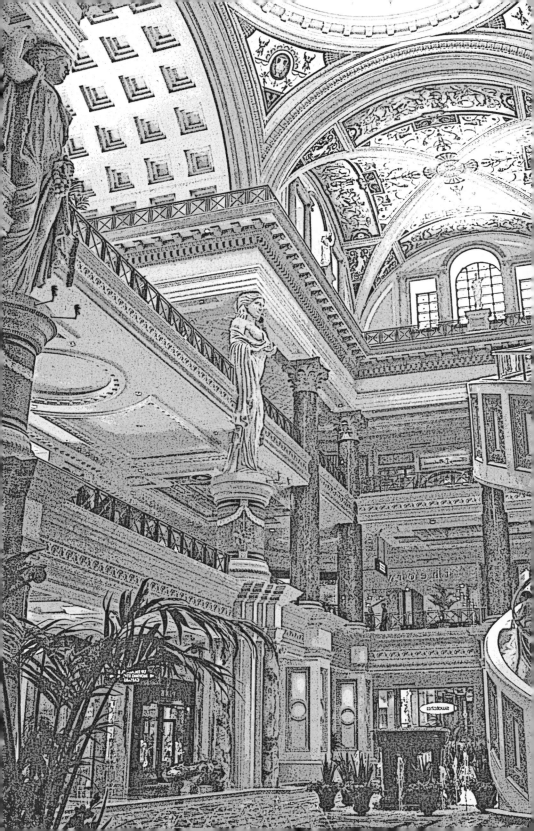

3

Housing

*Housing is not overly important . . . unless you are
tired of sleeping in your car.*

*C*ontrary to the quote above, housing is one of the most important items to be considered. It is your home away from home: a place to kick back and relax. It needs to be clean, safe, comfortable, and close enough to your work to be reasonably convenient.

Overview

For most, housing is a "show stopper" when selecting a staffing agency. If the agency cannot provide the housing you feel you need, choose another agency. After all, you're providing the funds for all of this by your employment. Don't forget that!

The agency should provide your housing directly, or give you a monthly payment (called a "stipend" or "housing allowance") so you can make your own arrangements.

Here is a brief description of the major housing scenarios you will encounter as a traveler:

* The agency provides your housing including a complete furnishings package. They pay all costs and arrange any installations required. The housing is in the agency's name. You never see any bills and may not know (or care) how much the housing costs. The housing management performs maintenance as required.

* The agency provides your housing including at least a partial furnishings package. They pay the rent and the major utilities such as power, gas, etc., but you may be responsible for some costs such as the monthly telephone or TV cable bill. You may also be responsible to coordinate their installation. You provide some of the furnishing such as linens, pots and pans, and perhaps a TV. The housing is in the agency's name. Only those bills that you arrange are in your name. The housing management performs all maintenance for the unit.

* You choose to receive a monthly stipend from the agency in lieu of them providing housing. You are responsible for locating your housing and paying all deposits and costs associated with it. Everything is in your name. The agency is not legally involved in any way. The housing management performs maintenance as required.

* You choose to receive a monthly stipend and provide your own housing via some form of recreational vehicle (RV). You are responsible for all costs including maintenance of the unit.

Whether the agency is paying for your housing directly or you are receiving a stipend, just about any housing option you can think of is a possibility. This includes apartments, condos, rental houses, extended stay motels, and RV motor homes and trailers. Living with a friend or relative in the area is sometimes an option as well. But hopefully you won't be living in your car!

Insight

And don't be shy about your housing. If you arrive and find it truly unacceptable notify your recruiter immediately. If the problem can not be corrected you should be moved to another apartment or apartment complex. You may need to stay in a motel, paid for by your agency, until corrections can be made or other suitable housing can be located.

Here are some general housing issues:

Security. You need to feel safe and secure. If you are to be housed in an apartment, try to avoid the ground level. Look for security features such as guarded, gated entrances to the complex, building security requiring a pass card or security code, security cameras, and dead bolt locks on your apartment doors. Always lock your vehicle and do not leave money and valuables visible.

Maintenance. Your housing should be clean and properly maintained. Housing management should resolve issues in a reasonable amount of time. No one wants to live in a dump!

Noise. If you have lived in a private home in a quiet neighborhood, you are in for some adjustment. Even if you have the best apartment in the nicest area, living in close proximity to many others requires tolerance and flexibility.

Insight

For us the townhouse configuration is the best. It maximizes living space and best of all no one is above you stomping around! If you cannot find a townhouse, try to live in a top floor apartment. It's harder to move in and out, and carry groceries but at least it will be quieter.

Understand your cost responsibility. Be sure you understand what items, if any, you are responsible for. (We'll discuss this in detail when we talk about the different forms of apartments.) As mentioned previously, your agency may expect you to pay for TV cable and telephone service, and perhaps to coordinate their installation. Just be sure you understand who is responsible for what.

Deposits. Your agency should pay all deposits if they provide your housing. The exceptions may be any utilities you are responsible for and any pet deposits that may be required. Like everything else, responsibility for deposits is negotiable. For instance our agency has always paid our pet deposits.

Parking. The apartment complex may have different parking options. Some may entail additional cost. On one assignment our apartment complex had free open parking, but also had rows of carport spaces you could rent for $10 each per month. Prior to arriving, check with the apartment manager to see what is available and at what cost.

> **Insight** *Be sure to investigate parking costs and availability in large cities prior to signing your contract. It can cost several hundred dollars per month. If so, this needs to be part of your negotiated pay package. For instance, it cost $450/month to park in downtown Boston in 2006.*

Proximity to work. Travel time to work can be an issue, especially if you have to take call. Access to public transportation can sometimes be a plus. When you first arrive, take a practice run to your facility and see if it is close enough. If not, you may need to move.

Laundry. Laundry issues are often overlooked by the traveler until they arrive and begin their assignment. Be sure to ask how laundry is handled. Is a washer and dryer inside the apartment, down the hall, in a different building, non-existent? If your agency does not have the information, call the housing manager to get the details.

> ⚡*Insight*⚡ On our first assignment we thought it was wonderful to
> have a washer and dryer in each apartment until the guy
> above us decided to wash at 12:30 am. He vibrated the
> whole building until he finished about 3:00 am!
>
> Urban settings can also be challenging. In Boston we had to cart our laun-
> dry about 1/4 of a mile to the laundromat. We could have signed up for a
> laundry service but we saw how they wash clothes: by stuffing as many as
> they could in the washer, packing them in with a stick. No thanks.

Pets. We have mentioned this briefly before. If you travel with a pet,
you may have to accept slightly lower rated housing. Many higher
end apartments will not allow pets. Some may exclude dogs weigh-
ing over 40 pounds or certain breeds of aggressive dogs. And, again,
there could be a special deposit or additional monthly charge for your
pet. This is a negotiation point with your agency.

Apartment or Condo Provided by the Agency

Most travelers prefer this form of housing. They like the idea of not
having to find housing themselves. Anyone who has rented an apartment knows the hassle of finding a good complex close to work and
in a good part of town. Paying all those deposits along with coordi-
nating installation for such things as telephone and TV cable service
can be a real pain!

Many agencies work with "apartment finders". These companies specialize in placing professionals on short term assignments. They often
contract with other local companies to provide a "furnishings package" including such things as furniture, linens, pots and pans, etc.
They will use the criteria provided by your agency regarding maximum cost allowed and your personal situation, such as pets, how
close you need to be to your workplace, etc. The apartment finder
will locate the best possibilities and give your agency the options.
Given the circumstances, there could be only one or several options

from which to choose. Your agency will then provide you with the details. This should include the size, location, directions to get there, and the name and phone number of the manager. Some apartment complexes have a web site which shows the apartment floor plans and usually has representative photos. Once you have signed your work contract and tell your agency the housing appears to be acceptable, they will sign the lease and arrange payment to the housing management.

There are three forms of the private apartment: corporate, furnished, and partially furnished or unfurnished.

Corporate apartment. This is the top of the line in apartment living. It is a private, fully furnished, and at least modestly decorated apartment provided at no cost to you. It should have at least one bedroom. It is equipped with the normal things you would find in your home such as a fully equipped kitchen with dishes, glasses, pots, pans, utensils, microwave, can opener, refrigerator, dishwasher, etc. The bed should be reasonably sized, and the bedroom should contain a dresser and at least minimal storage space. You should find a full compliment of sheets, pillow cases, pillows, towels and wash cloths. The living area should be large enough and contain enough furniture for you to be comfortable. It should be clean and in good condition. There should be enough tables and lamps. All utilities, a TV with at least a basic cable package, and phone service (excluding long distance) should be provided at no cost to you.

The idea of corporate housing is to arrive, open the door, and find everything you need already there (except food and personal need items). Your agency makes all the arrangements and you should never receive any bills or statements.

Furnished apartment. This is similar to the corporate apartment with the exception that you may have to provide some of the items yourself. It should contain the necessary furniture items, but may not contain linens, pots and pans, a TV or phone. You may have to arrange for TV cable and telephone service and may have to pay for them yourself. Be sure you understand exactly what will be provided. Just as with the corporate apartment, the agency should contract directly with the apartment complex and you should never see any bills except for those services you are expected to arrange and pay for separately.

Partially furnished or unfurnished apartment. Many travelers prefer to take some of their personal items on assignment. They may want their own bed, dishes, pictures, even their favorite couch or chair. Of course, it is more effort to move in and out when changing assignments. But if you plan to be at the same location for an extended time, it can help you feel more at home. Your agency can reduce or perhaps even eliminate the furnishings package they would rent for you each month. The savings may then be reflected in your paycheck as extra income.

Shared Apartment

Some agencies want you to share an apartment with one or more travelers while on assignment. They will allow you to have a private apartment only if you pay the difference, or if you are on a "select assignment". If this meets your life style, that's fine. If not, choose another agency to travel with. The shared apartment normally falls into either the corporate or the furnished category depending on what items and services are provided. Again, be sure you understand what your agency will be providing and your responsibility, if any.

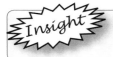 *And be sure to ask where the bathroom is. On a shared apartment it might be down the hall and serving many others!*

Using Extended Stay Motels

If your agency has placed several travelers at a facility, they probably have a good idea about the housing in the area. If not, you may want to be housed temporarily in an extended stay motel until you feel more confident about the choices in the area. Some travelers always insist on this option for the first week or two. This gives them time to examine the housing the agency has suggested and explore other options in the area that may be more desirable, yet still affordable. Check with the front desk and be sure your agency has given them their credit card for room payment. They may require yours as well to cover any incidentals.

> *Insight*
>
> *We lived in an extended stay suite during our entire assignment in Alaska. It had two bedrooms, two baths, three TV's, a full kitchen, maid service three times a week, laundry down the hall, and a spectacular view of the mountains. Not bad!*

Housing Stipend

As mentioned earlier, you can receive a stipend as an alternative to your agency providing housing. Stipends work well for those using RV's, or that stay with friends or relatives. They also work well for travelers willing to accept the added burden of finding their own housing in exchange for potentially more money per month. Your agency will often act as if the stipend amount is firm, but it is actually a negotiated monthly amount paid directly to you and is tax-free, if you qualify. It just can not exceed the IRS limit for lodging in your assignment area (more about this in Chapter 5 describing tax advantage programs). The stipend is prorated per pay period or paid as a single monthly amount. You then make all the housing arrangements. If you find housing for less than the stipend, you pocket the difference. If you can't find housing at the stipend rate call your recruiter and see if they can increase the amount. Many travelers and even some agencies use www.craigslist.org and other web resources to locate potential housing.

Your stipend should be at least equivalent to the amount your agency would spend on housing for you, although this is sometimes difficult to verify. Actually, the stipend should be **more** than the agency would have spent because they avoid the hassle of finding and setting up your housing. That should be worth something to them!

You can estimate the stipend amount in several ways. Your agency may use one or more apartment complexes to house travelers on assignment. Ask your agency where you would stay if you took their housing option and how much it costs them. If they are reluctant to discuss costs, call the manager of the complex and see if they will tell you how much they charge your agency. Another method is to call several apartment complexes in the area that provide corporate or furnished housing and ask their cost. Ask if short term leases are available and if there is a premium involved for them. If no such apartments exist locally you can estimate the cost by asking the apartment rental rate, and then by calling a rental furnishing business that specializes in providing for homes and apartments. Add a little more for cable TV and local telephone service and you should be close to the minimum stipend rate. Again, you can consult resources on the web to see what is available in the local area.

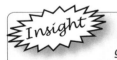 *Many travelers simply ask for the maximum lodging amount allowed by the IRS for that area rather than negotiating a stipend figure with the agency.*

Be careful if you plan to use a stipend to get your own apartment. Your agency has certain advantages when it comes to leasing. As an established business, they have more clout to negotiate short term leases. True, they may pay a premium per month, but this allows somewhat of an open-ended arrangement with the apartment complex. Your agency pays for only the time required. If you are there for

13 weeks, that's what they schedule. If you suddenly extend, they call and extend the lease as required. As an individual, the apartment complex may not be willing to give you the same leeway. You may be tied to incremental leases such as six months or a year, with a penalty involved if not completed.

Insight

And suppose you arrive for your assignment, sign the lease, pay the deposits, and suddenly your work contract is cancelled. If your agency made all the housing arrangements they will be stuck with this nightmare, not you!

RV'ing It

Some prefer to take their home with them. Traveling by recreational vehicle (RV) is a popular alternative to having your agency provide housing. The stipend is used to recoup operating expenses, campground fees, and payments on the RV. Many enjoy the casual lifestyle that RV parks generally provide and enjoy camping along the way to and from assignments. There are a number of books, magazines, atlases, and web resources available to aid in planning your trips and finding RV parks and campgrounds. Trailer Life, Woodall's, and Frommer's publish campground directories. Some join Good Sam Club, Escapees, or other groups that offer discounts, trip planning, etc. A book called "The Next Exit: USA Interstate Highway Directory ..." by Mark Watson lists service stations, motels, and restaurants at the Interstate exits. Also, Delphi has a discussion forum called "Nurses on Wheels".

The three major categories of RV for the traveler are the motorhome, the trailer, and the fifth wheel. Slide-in campers and pop-up trailers are other options but are generally not considered practical for long term living.

The motorhome is a self contained unit having the living area and driving vehicle on the same chassis. The Class A motorhomes are the larger bus-looking vehicles. The Class B motorhomes are small motorhomes built on van chassis while the Class C motorhomes start with a cutaway chassis with a van or truck front end. They usually have a section extending over the top of the driving cab.

A trailer is a living unit that attaches to your vehicle, normally a pick-up truck, at the rear bumper. It connects via a trailer ball and hitch. It is recommended to have a weight distribution bar and an anti-sway bar. They help distribute the weight more evenly to your vehicle and add sway control to help counter high winds.

The fifth wheel is also a trailer. However, it attaches to a truck with a special hitch that sits in the bed directly over the back wheels. This system adds stability in cross winds and allows your truck to pull a heavier load.

If you are into snowmobiling, motorcycles, or ATV's, you may consider a "toy hauler". Along with a living area these units have a special enclosed cargo area at the back for storage.

To be comfortable on the road, consider a unit that is at least 30 to 35 feet long. Longer if you think you need the room. When choosing a trailer or a fifth wheel, be sure your vehicle is capable of towing it safely. This often requires a diesel pickup. Be sure to have a good towing package with proper connections for lights and a trailer braking system.

So how much can you expect to pay for an RV? As you might expect the Class A motorhomes are the most expensive, costing $100,000 to $500,000 and up. Some cost more than a million. The Class B motorhomes are usually priced in the $60,000 to $100,000 range while Class C motorhomes often fall into the range of $70,000 to $200,000 with some units as high as $300,000.

Trailers cost between $20,000 and $35,000 with some models priced about $50,000. Fifth wheels tend to be a little heavier and a little more costly. They generally cost between $30,000 and $70,000 with some models over $100,000. Toy haulers can be found in just about every category and are in those same price ranges.

When shopping for an RV visit as many dealers as you can. Get their brochures and look up the manufacturer's web sites for additional sizes and floor plans that were not at the dealers' site. The manufacturer's web sites should have a dealer locator. This allows you to find the dealers closest to you that carry the models of interest.

Trailers and fifth wheels have two major types of construction: wood or aluminum framing. Aluminum is stiffer and lighter. It takes the swaying and vibration of the road better than wood framing, but as you might expect it costs more. Choose a unit with enough water tank capacity for your needs and with at least thirty amp electrical service. Fifty amp capacity is even better and becoming the standard. If you plan to stay in a cold climate, talk to your dealer about installing a winterizing kit. Many RV's come equipped with that option from the manufacturer.

RV'ing can be fun and rewarding. But it can also generate some problems. You may have to choose assignments based on campground and trailer park locations and availability. Many campgrounds are closed during the winter in the colder regions of the country. Even in warmer months, you may have trouble staying within a reasonable distance of your work in or near large urban areas. Being subject to call can be a real drawback. Having to live within 30-45 minutes of your job can severely restrict your options. Also, some RV parks limit the size they will accept. Sometimes 35 feet is the maximum length. Some limit your length of stay to as little as 14 days. Don't just consider campgrounds. There may be some nice trailer parks in the vicinity that accept RV's.

Your RV can be considered as a second home. The interest cost associated with financing your RV could be tax deductible. If your RV is your full time home and you do not have a "permanent home" under IRS rules, you will be classified as an itinerant worker. Reimbursements for housing may no longer qualify as tax-free. Please check with your tax advisor if you think this may be a problem for you.

> *Insight*   Buying an RV can be a large investment. If you are considering becoming a traveler and wish to pursue the RV option, I suggest you complete at least a couple of assignments taking the apartment option from your agency to be sure traveling is right for you. If you still feel you want to travel in an RV, make the investment and go for it!

Buying an RV – Our Personal Story

We had always taken the corporate housing option. But throughout the summer of 2007 we discussed buying an RV for traveling. Being close to retirement we decided to buy one and pay for it prior to actually retiring.

Buying an RV can be an interesting experience. If you think the markup on new automobiles is significant, you are in for a real awakening when it comes to an RV! In December of 2007 we purchased a 35 foot long 5th wheel. We negotiated a price 42% less than the MSRP. This was our strategy.

We made a short list of the things we felt we truly wanted, such as a king size bed, space for a stackable washer and dryer, the entertainment center had to be easily visible from every part of the living area, and a length of 35 feet or less to get into at least most of the places we wanted to visit. We also wanted to buy the new 2008 model to get the latest innovations available.

Next we visited all the dealers we could in our home area to get an idea of the models that would meet our criteria and the prices involved. Because the dealers do not have all the brands and models available on their lot, we checked online and looked at almost literally every floor plan from every manufacturer. Once we decided on a brand and floor plan, we found those dealers by going online to the manufacturer's web site. We called the dealers in our region to see if they had the exact floor plan we wanted. If they did, we made it clear that we were going to buy that RV from someone in the region within one week and we wanted their lowest price.

We began serious discussions with the dealer willing to provide the model we wanted at the lowest price. In addition to verifying the options and purchase price, we also negotiated the financing as part of the deal. We made it clear that we were not leaving our home driveway until all the cost details for both the RV and the financing were known. This way we felt we got the lowest competitive financing rate. We gave the dealer a few personal details over the phone. They ran the necessary credit check, gave us the terms, and e-mailed an itemized list of the exact final cost.

Once we were satisfied we gave the dealer a credit card deposit for $500 to hold the RV. We verified that this in no way obligated us and if things were not as advertised when we arrived our deposit would be returned and the deal cancelled. At the dealership, we verified all the options on the RV and all the financing details. We had to drive 400 miles to pick it up but the savings made it worthwhile.

Notes

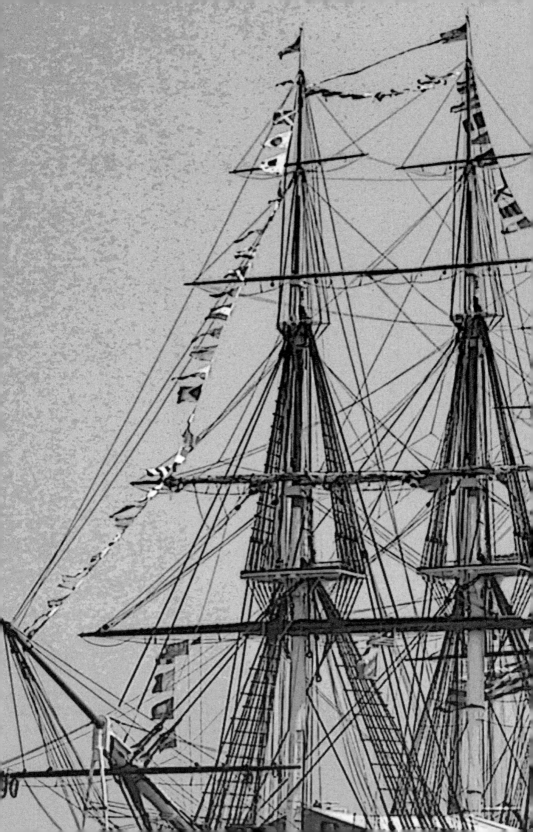

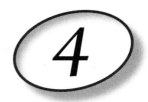

Benefits

*There's nothing "free" about your benefits.
It all comes out of the bill rate, which you earn.*

*A*long with housing, benefits are also one of the most important issues to travelers. Here's a look at . . .

What's Available

The benefits offered by agencies vary widely. Agency web sites and magazine advertisements can produce a "laundry list" of items offered. No agency offers them all, so you have to decide which are most important when choosing your agencies. Here's a list I was able to generate:

* Weekly pay
* Direct deposit
* Double pay for overtime
* Guaranteed pay
* Paid time off

- Bonuses:
    - Sign-on
    - Completion
    - Extension
    - Referral
    - Loyalty
- 401(k) plan (with employer match)
- Insurance:
    - Health
    - Dental
    - Prescription
    - 125 Cafeteria Plan
    - Vision
    - Life
    - Disability insurance (short and long term)
    - Professional liability
- License reimbursement
- Tuition and CEU assistance
- Bereavement pay
- Advanced certification assistance
- Free income tax preparation
- 24/7/365 accessibility
- Free telephone calling cards, discount cards, etc

And one agency advertised they even do your laundry!

Benefit Details

Weekly pay. Most agencies will pay you on a weekly basis, even though they do not receive payment from the facility that often. Facilities are notorious for being slow to pay. The agency pays you from their corporate bank account and then recoups the money from the facility as it comes in. Some agencies may pay you every two weeks or even monthly, but weekly pay is the norm.

Direct deposit. In this day and age every agency should provide direct deposit and every traveler should take advantage of it. The security issues caused by sending paychecks through the mail should be avoided. Have your pay deposited directly into a bank account in your home area. This helps prove you have business ties to your permanent home. Access your money via the cash back option at local stores, or through ATM's while on assignment. Be sure your bank is a member of the FDIC. We'll talk more about these issues in Chapter 12.

Double pay for overtime. The normal overtime pay rate is time and one half but some assignments may pay double for overtime. This is usually only available for assignments in highly specialized areas or for hard to fill vacancies.

Guaranteed pay. Many travelers insist their contracts contain a clause guaranteeing their weekly hours. If any shifts are cancelled or shortened by the facility, the traveler still receives their full weekly pay. This prevents the facility from using them PRN and assures them of the income they expected when they accepted the assignment.

Paid time off. A few agencies offer a paid vacation after you have worked with them for a year or so. If you qualify they may give you a week's pay or more. If you change assignments and agencies often you will have difficulty qualifying for this benefit.

Bonuses: sign-on, completion, extension, referral, loyalty. An agency may offer you a sign-on bonus if you will accept an assignment with them. You may need a specialty in high demand, or be willing to take a hard to fill vacancy.

A completion bonus may be available after successfully completing an assignment. Sometimes there are a total number of hours to be completed during the contract. If you miss some time for any reason and cannot make it up, you may not qualify for the bonus.

Some receive a bonus if they extend an assignment. If a facility has an acceptable traveler in place they no doubt prefer them to stay rather than trying to find another traveler to take the assignment.

Agencies often advertise referral bonuses. If you recommend a traveler who then completes an assignment with that agency, you get a bonus. It is usually in the $500 to $1000 range but can be more depending on the specialty. You do not have to work for the agency to refer someone to them and collect the bonus.

The loyalty bonus is used to reward travelers who have stayed with the agency for a significant time. The rules to qualify can vary for each agency.

401(k) plan (with employer match). Your agency should offer a 401(k). (If not, find another agency!). And even better, they may offer to match a portion of your contributions. This is free money so make an effort to contribute at least enough to qualify for the match. (More about your 401(k) in Chapter 13.)

Health insurance: medical, dental, prescription, vision. Health insurance is probably the benefit travelers are most concerned with. If this is important to you, choose an agency with an adequate plan and be sure you understand the coverage, cost, deductible, and the policy on pre-existing illness. The plans may include at least some coverage for dental, prescriptions, and vision issues. Be sure to ask your recruiter the rules for continuing your coverage during time off between assignments.

125 Cafeteria Plan. Occasionally you will find an agency that offers a 125 Cafeteria Plan as their health insurance coverage. This is an approved IRS program dealing with medical and medically related issues. Employee contributions are allowed on a pre-tax basis. There are four basic forms of the plan:

The first is the simplest form of cafeteria plan. It enables participants covered by a contributory medical plan to have their contributions changed from after-tax to pre-tax dollars.

The second form is like the first, except that participants are given a choice of various medical plans. Each plan has a different level of coverage and requires a different employee contribution.

Another allows participants to contribute to one or more flexible spending accounts as a supplement to their medical plan coverage. They can withdraw the money as needed to cover approved costs.

The last form is an employer credit plan. The employer provides each participant with a number of credits that are usually enough to enable the participant to purchase at least a minimum level of benefits without extra cost to them. The participant can spend the credits on a more expensive benefit plan and/or contribute them to one or more flexible spending accounts.

As with other health care coverage, be sure you understand the options and costs involved, and ask about the policy for continuing your coverage between assignments.

Other insurance: life, disability, professional liability. Agencies sometimes pay the complete cost for a certain level of life insurance. If you want more coverage you pay the difference. Disability insurance (short and long term) may also be available. Agencies sometimes have an umbrella policy that provides free professional liability insurance for all their travelers.

Licensure reimbursement. Licenses are expensive to acquire and renew. In my opinion, your agency should reimburse you for the costs incurred for the license used while on assignment and pay you back if you have to renew it while on assignment.

Tuition and CEU assistance. Your agency may be willing to defray some or all of the costs for tuition, and for any CEU's required to renew your licenses.

Bereavement pay. Paid time off and some travel assistance may be available.

Advanced certification assistance. Some agencies are willing to pay the fees associated with getting and maintaining advanced certification.

Free income tax preparation. Tax preparation can be difficult. Given the issues involved in traveling it is recommended you hire a qualified tax advisor. Agencies will sometimes assist you by paying all, or reasonable amount, toward this service.

24/7/365 accessibility. Almost every agency will have a staffer on call for emergency needs.

Free telephone calling cards, discount cards, etc. Other perks may include phone calling cards, discount cards for local merchants, and yes, even laundry money!

Health Insurance Between Assignments

It is not unusual to find travelers that seldom extend their contracts. They like the variety of travel and experience. Others may stay longer by way of contract extensions. In any case the life of a traveler can entail changing agencies and assignment locations often (if for no other reason than to maintain tax-free status with the IRS).

Some travelers do not participate in their agency's health plan. They may be covered through private insurance or through a plan carried by their spouse. If this is the case, coverage between assignments is not a problem for you.

If you participate in your agency's health plan, there may be gaps in your coverage between assignments. Your agency may continue your coverage spanning short periods while they are trying to place you in your next assignment. However if you take extended time off, chances are your agency will not provide coverage for that period. So what do you do? Many turn to . . .

The **C**onsolidated **O**mnibus **B**udget **R**econciliation **A**ct. Wow, now that's a mouthful! You can almost guess from the name that this is Federal Government legislation . . . and you would be right. Congress passed the COBRA health benefits provisions in 1986. It provides health coverage at group rates to certain former employees, spouses, former spouses, retirees, and dependent children. The coverage is temporary and only available when your other coverage is lost due to certain "qualifying events" defined in the law. COBRA is normally more expensive than your agency's health plan (your agency will probably not contribute to the COBRA premium), but may be cheaper than individual private insurance. The law generally covers health plans offered by private sector companies with 20 or more employees. However, COBRA also applies to employee organizations, and to state and local governments.

To be eligible for coverage you must have been enrolled in your agency's plan while you worked for them and their health plan must continue in effect for those employees remaining with the agency. Coverage via COBRA is available if a qualifying event occurs that would cause you to lose your agency's coverage.

Here are the qualifying events from the Department of Labor Employee Benefits Security Administration web site http://www.dol.gov/ebsa (November 2008):

"Qualifying Events for Employees:

Voluntary or involuntary termination of employment for reasons other than gross misconduct

Reduction in the number of hours of employment

Qualifying Events for Spouses:

Voluntary or involuntary termination of the covered employee's employment for any reason other than gross misconduct

Reduction in the hours worked by the covered employee

Covered employee's becoming entitled to Medicare

Divorce or legal separation of the covered employee

Death of the covered employee

Qualifying Events for Dependent Children:

Loss of dependent child status under the plan rules

Voluntary or involuntary termination of the covered employee's employment for any reason other than gross misconduct

Reduction in the hours worked by the covered employee

Covered employee's becoming entitled to Medicare

Divorce or legal separation of the covered employee

Death of the covered employee"

If you are no longer eligible for continued coverage through your agency, they must notify their plan administrator within 30 days. The plan administrator then has 14 days to send you an election notice allowing you to continue healthcare coverage under COBRA. You then have 60 days to decide if you want COBRA coverage. If so, you have 45 days after electing COBRA to pay your first premium. COBRA will cost more since you are now responsible for the entire premium plus a 2% administration fee. The first payment must cover the period from the date of COBRA election retroactive to the date you lost coverage. If you waive COBRA coverage during the election period, you can revoke the waiver, but you must do so before the period expires. Coverage under COBRA begins on the date the coverage from your agency's plan ends and normally lasts a maximum of 18 months. In the case of disability, an additional 11 months of coverage is available. However you will need a ruling from the Social Security Administration stating you became disabled within the first 60 days of COBRA coverage, and you must send the plan a copy of the ruling. All this must be accomplished before the original 18 months of coverage has expired. Under certain qualifying events, such as an employee's death, a divorce, or legal separation, a beneficiary may be permitted to receive a total of 36 months of coverage.

Converting Benefits to Cash

Your agency may offer benefits you do not need. If so, they may be willing to give you the equivalent amount they would pay out as extra income on your paycheck.

For example, if you provide your own health coverage your agency may give you the same amount they give their employees for their premium contribution. Another option is for the agency to give you a lump sum payment up to a certain limit to cover, or help cover, your medical premiums with another carrier.

Insight — *Be sure your agency deposits the money as a separate item per pay period or monthly so you can be sure you receive it. For instance, if they agree to give you $200 per month they would have spent on your health insurance premium, be sure this extra $200 appears in your pay as a distinct item. Don't allow them to say it is simply mixed in with your other tax-free reimbursements. You may never receive it!*

Notes

Notes

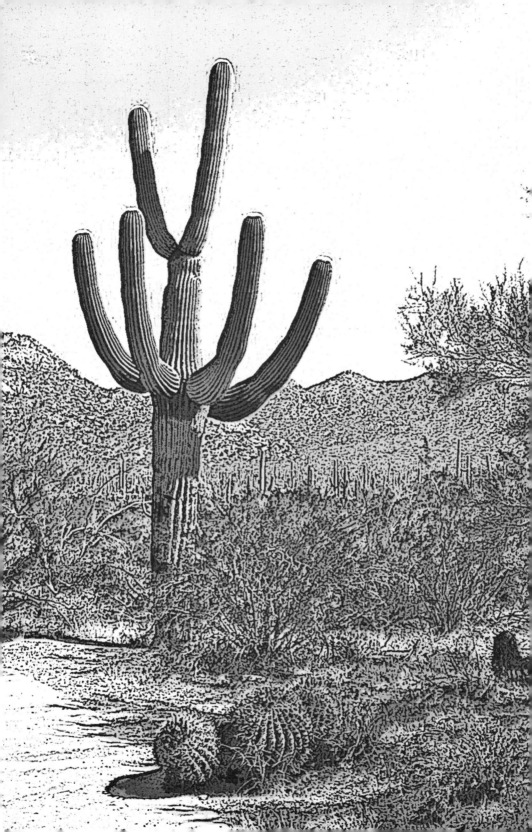

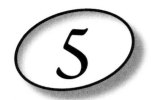

Tax Advantage Programs

Delaying the Tax Man is like cheating Death.
Both eventually win . . . but hopefully not today.

I tuned into a web discussion forum recently and saw a posting from an agency advertising a travel assignment paying forty eight dollars an hour. Forty eight dollars an hour! As a permanent staffer have you ever made that kind of money? You may have heard travelers receive a large hourly wage, say $40, $50, perhaps even $60 per hour. Do they really receive that? The answer is probably "yes". But to get the whole story you need to understand . . .

Combined Rates

Actually, permanent staffers make more per hour than they think. In addition to their hourly wage, they receive vacation time, sick leave, the facility may pay all or part of their health insurance premiums, etc. If you took the cost of those benefits and converted them to an equivalent hourly rate and then added it to the hourly wage you would have a **combined rate** (often called a blended rate). In other words the combined rate consists of your taxable hourly wage and all your benefits rolled into one hourly wage figure. For a qualified traveler the combined rate is an hourly amount that includes the hourly wage, benefits, **and tax-free reimbursements.**

How Tax Advantage Programs Work

Tax advantage programs are allowed under IRS rules. Travelers can receive tax-free reimbursements if they have a permanent home and accept temporary assignments that are far enough from home to prevent commuting (more about this in Chapter 6 on taxes). A portion of your pay package is taxable and a portion is tax-free. Agencies use one of two methods to produce the allocation between the two.

Total hourly wage method. This is what we have discussed so far. Wages, benefits, and tax-free reimbursements are rolled into one combined hourly rate the agency quotes you. From there you begin allocating a portion of this total amount for benefits and tax-free items. If you want per diem and a car allowance, those costs are converted to an hourly wage and subtracted from the total hourly amount. If you want health coverage, your portion of the premium is converted to an hourly wage and subtracted from the total. Once all your benefit and tax-free items are subtracted, you are left with your true taxable hourly wage. And of course this will be substantially lower than the original rate quoted by the agency. You still get all the money of the original hourly quote but a portion has now been reallocated to various other items. There is some latitude to vary the allocation to suit your needs. For instance, if you want to increase your tax-free portion then your taxable wage can be reduced accordingly, within reason. You just can't receive more in tax-free reimbursements than the IRS allows for that area, and the IRS wants to see an appropriate taxable hourly wage for your specialty and assignment area.

Here's a simplified example of an allocation. We'll use just the larger items to illustrate the process. Let's say your agency has quoted you a combined rate of $48 per hour. Your pay week consists of 40 hours. Of the $48 per hour, you would like the agency to furnish corporate housing and pay you the maximum for daily living expenses allowed by the IRS for your assignment area. You also want to participate in their health coverage plan. The agency determines the corporate housing package will cost $1700 per month. The maximum daily living allowance for the assignment area is $50 per day. Your portion of the health insurance premium is $250 per month. To find your true taxable hourly wage we must convert the items just mentioned to an equivalent hourly wage and subtract them from $48. By the way, there are 4.33 weeks per month (52 weeks per year divided by 12 months per year).

Housing cost: $1700 per month/4.33 = $392.61 per week
$392.61/40 hours per week = **$9.81 per hour**

Daily living allowance is paid for 7 days per week but allocated per your 40 hour work week.
$50 per day *7 days/40 hours = **$8.75 per hour**

Health insurance: $250 per month/4.33 = $57.74 per week
$57.74/40 hours = **$1.44 per hour**

Your real taxable hourly wage is:
$48 minus $9.81, $8.75, and $1.44 = $28 per hour

Keep in mind you still get the full $48 per hour. But $20 of it has been reallocated to tax-free items.

Separated items method. Rather than quoting a combined rate an agency may separate the items for you. This is easier for most to understand. In our simple example an agency would tell you the assignment carries a $28 per hour wage, corporate housing will be provided, the daily living allowance is $50 per day, and health insurance will cost $250 per month.

But don't forget that everything is negotiable! Depending on your situation and negotiating skill, you might be able to bump up that hourly rate or reallocate other items to your liking! Again, just don't exceed the IRS limits on tax-free reimbursements for your assignment area.

Tax-free Reimbursements

As mentioned, these items can increase your pay by 20% to 30%. Agencies are able to offer qualified travelers tax advantage programs approved by the IRS. Here are the items usually included:

Per diem. We will explore this topic in the next section. For now just note that per diem limits are based on government information published each year and are made up of two items: Lodging (your housing costs) and M&IE (daily living allowance for meals and incidental expenses). Your agency should pay for your housing while on assignment either directly to the housing manager or by a monthly stipend paid to you. The M&IE portion is reimbursement for daily living expenses such as food and personal items while on assignment away from your permanent home. Neither your lodging nor the M&IE can exceed their individual limits for your assignment area without generating a taxable event. Check with your agency and tax advisor if you have questions.

Travel costs. Your agency should pay for you to get to and from your assignment. If you are flying they should purchase the airline ticket and arrange for a rental car, if required.

If you are driving, the agency will normally use one of two payment methods to reimburse you: mileage rate or lump sum payment. The agency may calculate the mileage to the assignment and pay you a rate per mile. It should be based on the IRS mileage rate in effect at that time. The rate is examined each year and revised as required.

Your agency may choose to pay you a lump sum amount, say $400, to get to the assignment and the same amount at the end of the assignment to return home. Agencies may pay a reduced mileage rate but also give you a lump sum amount to help cover motel and other costs.

> **Insight** *The IRS mileage rate usually coincides with the GSA rate paid to Government employees while on travel. However, this is not always the case. In February 2008, the IRS rate was 50.5 cents per mile while the GSA rate was the older 48.5 cents per mile. Be sure to use the latest figure from the IRS.*

Car allowance. Some agencies pay for a rental car or allocate a portion of the tax-free payment to cover costs associated with a personal vehicle. It is a monthly reimbursement often prorated per week and based on the amount the agency would pay to rent the traveler a car for their assignment. It can be rolled into the per diem rate or paid as a separate item. Don't be too upset if your agency does not offer a car allowance as such. All you can legally receive is the maximum daily per diem rate allowed by the IRS. If you and your agency want to call a portion of it "car allowance", that's fine.

Equipment. Some specialty areas require unique equipment. Protective lead in radiology is a good example. Facilities usually provide protection but many travelers purchase their own. This helps assure a better fit and more comfort during longer cases. Your agency may agree to pay at least a portion of the cost as technology changes and newer equipment is available.

Parking. Depending on the assignment location, you may be able to negotiate additional reimbursements. Your agency may agree to pay for parking costs incurred in large urban areas where parking is at a premium. There may also be a cost for parking or shuttle service at your work facility.

License reimbursement. If you are required to obtain a new license for an assignment you should be reimbursed for all costs, including the cost of verification, fingerprints, transcripts, etc. Save your receipts to prove your costs. Your agency may be a little picky about this item. They may hesitate to reimbursement you if you already have a license in that state, even if you have never worked there.

Insight — *In my opinion your agency should reimburse you for the license the first time it is used in the state, no matter when it was obtained. After all if your specialty requires it, you can't work in the state without a license, can you? And you are actually doing the agency a favor by being prepared to work in several states when assignments are received. It is a cost required for employment and you should receive a one time reimbursement. Also, if you are working in a state when the license is due for renewal, I would expect reimbursement from the agency.*

IRS Per Diem Rates

Well, we've postponed it as long as we can. It's time to discuss one of the most confusing and misunderstood topics of traveling: per diem rates. We keep mentioning tax-free payments and the fact that they can not exceed IRS limits without incurring a taxable event. So just exactly what are these limits for different areas of the country?

Actually the per diem limits are not generated by the IRS. They are established and modified periodically by another Federal agency: the General Services Administration (GSA) Travel Management Policy. They establish the Federal Government per diem rates for the continental U.S. (CONUS). The per diem tables address two categories of tax-free reimbursement: **Lodging** and **M&IE** (meals and incidental expenses). These are the rates the Federal Government pays its employees while they are traveling on temporary duty assignments. So why are these important to you? The IRS accepts the GSA limits as the maximum allowed for those in the private sector that qualify for tax-free reimbursements while working temporarily away from home. Hopefully that's you!

The rates are based on cost data collected throughout the U.S. and are revised as required. They are published each year to coincide with the Federal Government's fiscal year which starts October 1 and ends on September 30 of the following year. The per diem rates are listed in IRS Publication 1542 *Per Diem Rates (For Travel Within the Continental United States)*. I suggest downloading a copy from the publications section of www.irs.gov. Keep in mind the Government can issue revisions at any time, so you may want to visit the IRS web site periodically throughout the year to be sure you have the latest information.

For example, IRS Publication 1542 (Rev. October 2008) *Per Diem Rates (For Travel Within the Continental United States)* would have the per diem rates for the period October 1, 2008 through September 30, 2009. The IRS has rules which apply to the transition from one fiscal year to another, so each edition includes the previous fiscal year's rates along with the new rates.

By the way, as if things are not confusing enough, the per diem rates for states and U.S. territories outside the continental U.S. (OCONUS) are established by the Department of Defense Per Diem Committee. These include the states of Alaska and Hawaii, and all U.S. territories such as Guam, Puerto Rico, and the Virgin Islands. To find these rates you can search for "DOD Per Diem Committee" to find their web site or, easier still, use a search string with the location name: for example "Hawaii per diem rate".

So let's see how to use the per diem rate tables. As an example let's use IRS Publication 1542 (Rev. October 2008) *Per Diem Rates (For Travel Within the Continental United States)*. There are four tables in each year's publication. Tables 1 and 2 are high-low tables for certain areas of the country. These are simplified tables a company may choose to use. Table 3 is the per diem information for the previous year in case an assignment spans from the previous year. But Table 4 lists the per diem tables for the latest fiscal year, so let's focus on it.

In our example, the opening paragraph of Table 4 states:

> "Note: The standard rate of $109 ($70 for lodging and $39 for M&IE) applies to all locations within the continental United States (CONUS) not specifically listed below or encompassed by the boundary definition of a listed point. However, the standard CONUS rate applies to all locations within CONUS, including those defined below, for certain relocation allowances. (See parts 302-2, 302-4, and 302-5 of 41 CFR.)"

This establishes the nationwide base rate for lodging and for M&IE for the 48 contiguous states for October 1, 2008 though September 30, 2009 as $70 per day for lodging and $39 per day for M&IE. By the way, per diem rates apply to each and every day you are on assignment, including weekends.

Only areas that are higher than this base nationwide rate are listed in the tables. These are called "high cost" areas. If your assignment area is not listed in the tables, and does not fall within a county or defined location in the tables, the maximum daily per diem is the nationwide rate of $70 for lodging and $39 for M&IE.

As an example, the maximum daily per diem rates for the high cost areas of the state of Montana from Publication 1542 (Rev. October 2008) are shown on the opposite page. As you can see, the maximum daily per diem for some high cost areas remain constant throughout the year while others vary.

Key City	County and/or Defined Location	Effective Dates	Lodging	M&IE	Total
Big Sky, West Yellowstone	Gallatin	1/1-6/30	$82	$49	$131
		7/1-8/31	107	49	(156)
		9/1-12/31	82	49	131
Butte	Silver Bow	All Year	80	44	124
Helena	Lewis and Clark	All Year	77	44	121
Missoula, Polson, Kalispell	Missoula, Lake, Flathead	1/1-5/31	84	44	128
		6/1-8/31	106	44	(150)
		9/1-12/31	84	44	128

The daily per diem rates for the Butte and Helena areas remain constant for the entire year. The rates vary in the Big Sky, West Yellowstone, Missoula, Polson, and Kalispell areas. They increase in the summer months probably due to tourism and seasonal migration. Also, notice the rate increase is seen mostly in the cost of lodging. The M&IE rates change very little. This is typical of areas that have changing rates throughout the year. The County and/or Defined Location is a general term. Here are two quotes from that same publication clarifying the issue:

"Per diem localities with county definitions shall include 'all locations within, or entirely surrounded by, the corporate limits of the key city as well as the boundaries of the listed counties, including independent entities located within the boundaries of the key city and the listed counties (unless otherwise listed separately).'"

"**Note:** Recognizing that all locations are not incorporated cities, the term 'city limits' has been used as a general phrase to denote the commonly recognized local boundaries of the location cited."

It is important to understand the term "County and/or Defined Location". Even if your assignment location is not listed as a high cost area, you may be eligible for a higher per diem rate if your assignment falls within the "defined location" of a high cost area.

If your assignment spans more than one time period in the tables, the rate at which you start usually carries through the entire assignment. However, this can be a negotiating point if your assignment will be in a high cost area and there will be a variation in per diem rates throughout your contract period.

The term "per diem" is sometimes misused. If your agency provides your housing as a separately paid item you will not receive a lodging portion. This is what they use to pay for your housing and you will not see it on your paycheck. (You may not even know how much they pay.) Your agency may refer to the M&IE portion you receive as "per diem", since this portion is what you will receive on your paycheck. Using Helena, Montana, from our example, if your "per diem" is within reason of $121 per day it is full per diem: consisting of your lodging and M&IE. If the "per diem" figure is closer to $44 per day it constitutes only the M&IE portion. The bottom line is the value of your housing (or stipend) can not exceed the maximum amount for lodging, and your M&IE can not exceed the maximum amount listed in the table, without the excess being subject to taxation. Check with your tax advisor on this.

If you are a seasoned traveler, go through your past assignment contracts and compare your tax-free reimbursements with the per diem tables for those areas. You may not have received the maximum rate allowed by the IRS. Why not? (Of course one explanation might be that the agency took advantage of you.)

Agencies must be competitive and the bill rate for that area may not have been able to support the full amount. So let's look at an example. Let's consider the highest rates for Phoenix from that same IRS publication. Assume you took an assignment there starting in January 2009. You can receive $160 per day for lodging and $59 per day for M&IE. Let's also assume you are being paid $28 per hour, work 40 hours per week, and the agency makes 20% profit. The required bill rate would be approximately:

```
$160perday*7days/40hrsperweek =  $28.00 per hour
  $59perday*7days/40hrsperweek =   10.33 per hour
                   Your wage =   28.00 per hour
             Total so far is $66.33 per hour
```

If the agency wants to make 20% profit, the $66.33 is 80% of the required bill rate. $66.33/0.80 = **$82.91** total bill rate. An agency with a bill rate this high may have trouble competing.

Let's take a quick look at our example using the low-end per diem rates for Phoenix during the summer. Lodging is $96 per day and M&IE is $59 per day.

```
$96perday*7days/40hrsperweek =  $16.80 per hour
$59perday*7days/40hrsperweek =   10.33 per hour
                 Your wage =   28.00 per hour
           Total so far is  $55.13 per hour
```

$55.13/0.80 = **$68.91** per hour bill rate. While this is lower than the $82.91, an agency may still have trouble competing with this rate.

You might be asking, "If agencies sometimes have trouble paying the maximum in the per diem tables, what real use are the tables?" Hopefully you **can** receive the maximum in your assignment area! If not, the tables can serve as a guide to help negotiate a reasonable amount for tax-free reimbursements, especially in high cost areas. For instance if the M&IE for an area is $50 and your agency offers you $35, it is probably too low. If they offer you something closer to $50 (say $46) it would be more in line.

Foregoing Tax Advantage Programs

Some travelers do not use tax advantage programs. Here are a few of the issues involved:

The traveler is not eligible for such a program. If a traveler does not qualify under IRS criteria, the usual tax-free items such as housing, daily living allowance, travel costs, etc., will be taxable. We'll discuss the eligibility for tax-free reimbursements in the next chapter on taxes.

Their agency does not offer a program. Believe it or not, some agencies do not offer a tax advantage program. They may cite a number of reasons but any agency serious about staying in business and expanding will have to offer such a program. There are simply too many travelers that wish to take advantage of it, and there are too many competing agencies already offering such a program.

The traveler chooses not to participate. Even if eligible, some travelers choose to pay taxes on all, or part, of their tax-free reimbursements. While many would consider them out of their mind, there is an argument to be considered. Social Security payments are based on taxable earnings for a 35 year period. By foregoing the tax advantage program, your taxable income will be higher, and thus your ultimate Social Security monthly benefit will be higher during your retirement years.

Insight — *While this concept is worthy of consideration, it is difficult to predict the amount of a future monthly benefit check given that Congress will eventually have to "fix" Social Security. We personally use tax advantage programs. By contributing to a 401(k) and putting tax-free money to work in other ways, we feel we can outperform any increased monthly benefit that may occur by having all the income taxed.*

Notes

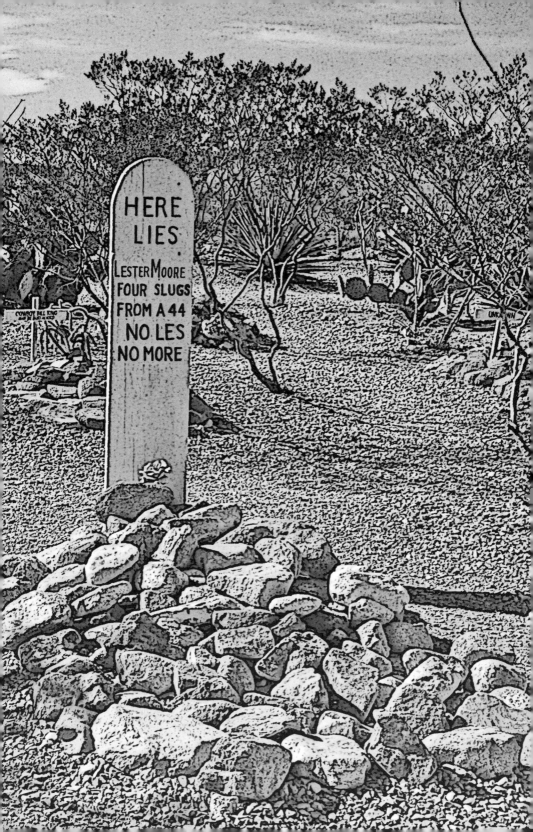

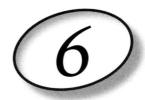

Taxes

*Anyone who enjoys paying taxes is in
dire need of medication.*

*A*pril 15th. Now that's a red letter day, isn't it? Who among us enjoys paying taxes? But as we have already seen, when it comes to paying taxes as a traveler there can be some . . .

Good News

Tax-free reimbursements can be some of the best news about traveling. Who doesn't want to make as much money as they can and legally reduce their tax burden as much as possible? Of course there is always that little catch phrase: "if you qualify". But if you do, a significant percentage of your income can be tax-free! So what does it take to prove to the IRS you are eligible for this tax-free money?

As a traveler your work can be very "fluid". Contracts are usually for 13 weeks. Sometimes they are extended. Sometimes you move on to another assignment or return home for awhile. You may work in only one state or several during the year. You may be on the road for many months or just a few, and your assignments may often take you far from home. Your income and tax situation can vary radically from year to year.

IRS Publication 463, *"Travel, Entertainment, Gift, and Car Expenses"*, sets the criteria for tax-free reimbursements. You can download a copy from the publications section at www.irs.gov. If you qualify under these guidelines, your reimbursements for the items we have mentioned previously (housing, daily living allowance, travel costs, etc,) will be exempt from taxation. There are several "speed bumps" that must be navigated to qualify for this advantage. The prevailing thought seems to be you must satisfy the following three conditions:

1. **You must maintain a permanent home.**

2. **Your assignments must be temporary in nature.**

3. **Your assignments must be far enough away from your permanent home to qualify for the IRS daily "sleep and rest" requirement.**

And of course the IRS interpretation of these conditions may not coincide with what you feel is fair and reasonable.

You Must Maintain a Permanent Residence

Here are a couple of important definitions:

Permanent residence. This is the physical place you call your home while you are away on assignment. It is where you have established business ties such as bank accounts, driver's license, car registration, doctor's appointments, and conduct a significant amount of personal business. You do not have to be a homeowner. Rental property such as an apartment can qualify. Your permanent home must be habitable. You cannot claim a post office box, a vacant piece of land, a storage building, or a storage building area as a permanent home.

Tax home. This is where the IRS says your regular place to conduct business is for tax purposes. The problem is it may not coincide with what you call your permanent home. Quoting from IRS Publication 463, *"Travel, Entertainment, Gift, and Car Expenses"* (2007):

> "Generally, your tax home is your regular place of business or post of duty, regardless of where you maintain your family home. It includes the entire city or general area in which your business or work is located. If you have more than one regular place of business, your tax home is your main place of business."

So, your goal should be to prove your permanent residence and your IRS tax home are one and the same.

If you work locally, live at your permanent residence most of the year, and take travel assignments only occasionally, proving your permanent residence is also your tax home should not be difficult. But suppose you spend much of your time on assignment away from home, returning only periodically to rest and work locally. And suppose you change assignment locations throughout the year. It may be more difficult to prove your main place of business for tax purposes is your permanent address. Again quoting from IRS Publication 463 (2007):

> "If you do not have a regular or main place of business because of the nature of your work, then your tax home may be the place where you regularly live."
>
> *"Factors used to determine tax home.* If you do not have a regular or main place of business or work, use the following three factors to determine where your tax home is.
>
> 1) You perform part of your business in the area of your main home and use that home for lodging while doing business in the area.

2) You have living expenses at your main home that you duplicate because your business requires you to be away from that home.

3) You have not abandoned the area in which both your historical place of lodging and your claimed main home are located; you have a member or members of your family living at your main home; or you often use that home for lodging.

If you satisfy all three factors, your tax home is the home where you regularly live. If you satisfy only two factors, you may have a tax home depending on all the facts and circumstances. If you satisfy only one factor, you are an itinerant; your tax home is wherever you work and you cannot deduct travel expenses."

Keep in mind that "business" activity is not just your work as a traveler. It is all aspects of your business life, such as banking, mortgage payments, doctor's appointments, purchasing a car, paying insurance premiums, repairs of all kinds, etc. Keep as many business activities tied to your permanent home location as possible. Here are some of the items that can help prove you have established and substantial business ties to your permanent home town area:

- A physical home address
- Home and car insurance, and repair bills
- Local bank checking and savings accounts
- Local utility bills
- Driver's license and car registration in your home state
- Local voter registration
- Local doctor and dentist services
- Local veterinarian services
- Home town volunteer and civic activities

And go ahead and throw in that old library card! The more proof the better!

Here are some things you can do to avoid generating confusion regarding your permanent residence:

* Avoid opening bank accounts while on assignment. Use your local home bank as much as possible. Banking online, direct deposit, bill paying options, and use of your ATM card can eliminate the need to open an account on the road and helps prove your ties to your permanent home.

* If possible, have all your mail (personal and professional) sent to your permanent home address and have it forwarded to your assignment location periodically.

* Keep your permanent address as your official billing address for all bills and credit cards.

* If you buy a car, boat, camper, trailer, etc, register it in your home state.

* You should always seek medical and dental treatment as required, but try to schedule routine checkups and elective procedures at home between assignments.

> **Insight** *Instead of using our home street address, we use a post office box in our home town as our permanent mailing address. The post office forwards our mail to our assignment location.*

Be careful if you plan to use the residence of a friend or family member as your permanent home address. My understanding is you must pay a reasonable amount of rent and the renter must claim that amount as income on their taxes. Check with your tax advisor to be sure. The last thing you need is for all of your tax-free money to suddenly be ruled taxable by the IRS.

Is Your Assignment "Temporary"?

Your assignment must be temporary to qualify for tax-free reimbursements. Again, some definitions:

Temporary job assignment. In general, an assignment lasting one year or less.

Indefinite job assignment. In general, an assignment that lasts, or is expected to last longer than one year. Here's what IRS Publication 463 (2007) says:

> "**Temporary assignment vs. indefinite assignment.** If your assignment or job away from your main place of work is temporary, your tax home does not change. You are considered to be away from home for the whole period you are away from your main place of work. You can deduct your travel expenses if they otherwise qualify for deduction. Generally, a temporary assignment in a single location is one that is realistically expected to last (and does in fact last) for one year or less.
>
> However, if your assignment or job is indefinite, the location of the assignment or job becomes your new tax home and you cannot deduct your travel expenses while there. An assignment or job in a single location is considered indefinite if it is realistically expected to last for more than one year, whether or not it actually lasts for more than one year.
>
> If your assignment is indefinite, you must include in your income any amounts you receive from your employer for living expenses, even if they are called travel allowances and you account to your employer for them."

And still quoting . . .

> "**Determining temporary or indefinite.** You must determine whether your assignment is temporary or indefinite when you start work. If you expect an assignment or job to last for one year or less, it is temporary unless there are facts and circumstances that indicate otherwise. An

assignment or job that is initially temporary may become indefinite due to changed circumstances. A series of assignments to the same location, all for short periods but that together cover a long period, may be considered an indefinite assignment."

The last sentence is an example of ambiguity sometimes encountered in tax publications. It is a judgment call as to how many assignments, how close together they can be, and how long they can extend, to still be defined as "temporary". If you work an assignment at the same location for over a year but have several contract breaks during the year, is this still a temporary assignment? How long do the breaks have to be? Confusion abounds among agencies and on web discussion forums. Your tax advisor should have an opinion on this.

Is Your Assignment Far Enough From Home?

For tax-free reimbursements, your assignments cannot be too close to your permanent home. From IRS Publication 463 (2007):

"You are traveling away from home if:

Your duties require you to be away from the general area of your tax home (defined later) substantially longer than an ordinary day's work, and

You need to sleep or rest to meet the demands of your work while away from home.

This rest requirement is not satisfied by merely napping in your car. You do not have to be away from your tax home for a whole day or from dusk to dawn as long as your relief from duty is long enough to get necessary sleep or rest."

My understanding is if you are able to commute to work, (whether you actually do or not) you are not far enough away from your home to qualify for tax-free reimbursements. Check with your tax advisor on this.

The "50 Mile Rule"

And while we are on this subject, let's mention a common misconception. Basically the "50 Mile Rule" states:

> You are eligible for tax-free reimbursements as long as your assignment is more than 50 miles away from your permanent residence.

The "50 Mile Rule" has been a common misunderstanding for a **long** time. As of this writing there is no basis for the rule in the IRS regulations. The regulations address the need to sleep and rest while away from home, but no minimum mileage is referenced. One can guess the "50 Mile Rule" may have originated as a general internal guide for businesses to determine if overnight accommodations might be required while traveling to allow proper rest after a full day of work. But again, you will have to satisfy the IRS guidelines as previously mentioned to qualify for tax-free reimbursements.

Record Keeping and Receipts

Many travelers keep extensive records for tax purposes. They record almost every cost associated with traveling. They save receipts of everything imaginable from grocery and gas to theater tickets. You may ask, "If the amount of tax-free reimbursements I receive covers my cost and is within the approved IRS limits, why do I need receipts and detailed records?" Tax advisors in general want to see as much evidence as possible. If nothing else, it supports you in case of an audit.

Also, it is possible for your costs to exceed the amount of tax-free reimbursements you receive. One example might be travel costs. Let's say your agency pays you $200 to get to an assignment but it actually costs you more. The excess may be a legitimate tax deduction. Another example might be your daily living allowance for meals and incidental expenses. Let's say you are in an area where the IRS allows $50 per day tax-free but your agency only pays you $40 per day. If you can justify expenses that exceed the $40 but are still under the allowed $50 they may be tax deductible.

Business supply stores have products for organizing your costs and saving receipts. Being well organized will help you prepare your taxes efficiently, avoid mistakes, and be ready if you are audited.

State Taxes

Probably the most difficult part of tax filing is handling state taxes. Working part of the year in one or more states away from your permanent home makes state tax filing confusing and sometimes difficult. As of this writing seven states have no personal income tax: Alaska, Florida, Nevada, South Dakota, Texas, Washington and Wyoming. Two others, New Hampshire and Tennessee, tax only dividends and interest. Your tax advisor can help you sort out your assignment locations, lengths of stay, and eligible reimbursements to be sure your state (and Federal) taxes are paid correctly.

Your agencies should withhold state and federal taxes correctly to be sure your situation is properly reflected on your W-2's.

Seek Expert Advice

Tax laws are constantly changing. Keeping up with the changes at the Federal level and for all fifty states is a difficult job. I am certainly not a tax expert and don't pretend to be. In fact, my experience is there are differences of interpretation among tax experts and also among agencies as to the proper handling of these issues. The wording found in the tax booklets published by the IRS and the state revenue departments is helpful but can be ambiguous and open to interpretation.

I suggest you find a qualified tax advisor that stays current and specializes in returns for travelers. Keep in mind there are no formal qualifications required to prepare taxes, so be careful. Don't be afraid to ask questions. Here are some of the things to look for in a tax advisor:

* Specializes in taxes for healthcare travelers, or at least for workers that travel frequently for months at a time.

* Prepares a lot of such tax returns, perhaps hundreds each year.

* Attends periodic educational presentations to remain current.

* Has been in business at least five years. The longer the better.

* Has survived audits and is willing to represent you, if required.

Interview the tax advisors and put them to the test. Ask some basic questions that you already know the answers to: such as what it takes to prove you have a tax home and how a temporary assignment is defined. Also, be sure to ask about their fee structure. If you feel uneasy about anything, move on. And if they quote the "50 Mile Rule" as criteria for tax-free reimbursement . . . run!

Insight — *Having a certification such as "CPA", while impressive, is no guarantee of extensive experience in a particular area. Be sure the tax advisor you choose has good knowledge and experience in the issues important to travelers.*

Notes

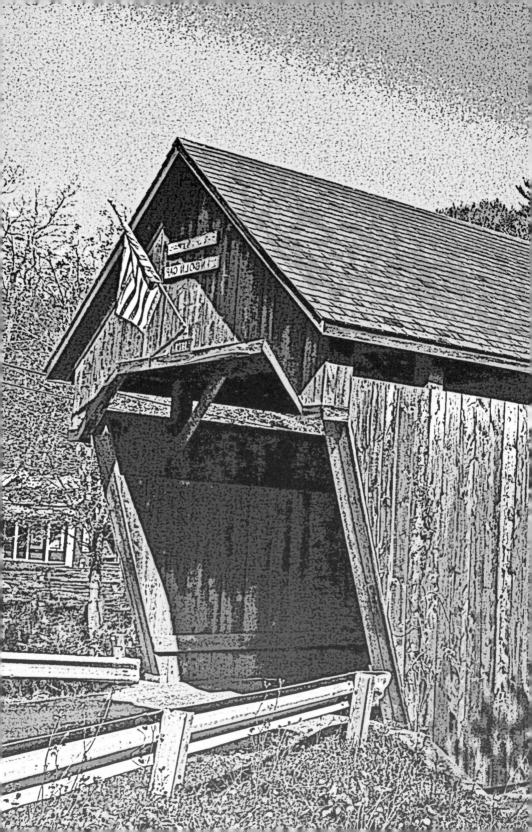

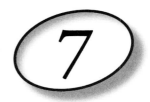

Your Contract

Trust is a wonderful thing.
(Just be sure to verify the details.)

O ne of the most surprising things we discovered when talking to travelers was how few of them understood the contracts they had signed. Many didn't care as long as they were being paid properly and things were running smoothly. It almost seemed to be a nuisance. Only if problems developed did they read their contract and then it was probably too late! Given this casual attitude, it is probably best to start this chapter by asking . . .

Why Are Contracts Necessary?

In a "perfect world" contracts would not be necessary. Everyone would be honest, forthright, and have a completely accurate understanding of all aspects of the agreement. Everyone would have the exact same interpretation of all portions of the agreement with no possibility of any misunderstanding.

Well, I think we have just discovered why we need contracts! Even well-meaning people can have differences of interpretation when reading a contract clause. Here's a simple example of how some wording may need clarification. Let's say a contract clause says:

"Private, furnished housing will be provided by the Agency."

Sounds simple enough? The agency will provide private housing that is furnished. But does the housing include utilities? Will they pay any deposits required? What does the word "furnished" mean? Will it include linens and kitchen items such as pots, pans, silverware, etc? You may be expecting **fully** furnished housing with all costs to be covered. But the agency may say "furnished housing" only refers to the actual housing structure containing basic furniture. They may expect you to pick up the other costs associated with apartment living. This could be a costly misunderstanding. You can see that more wording is required to clarify the situation.

> *Insight* *The written contract is the most important part of traveling. It governs all aspects of the assignment and is the only real, legal protection you have. Phone messages, personal notes, e-mail, testimony by others, etc, can be used as supporting evidence if problems arise. But if legal action is required, the contract clauses carry the primary weight in a court of law. Be sure they are complete and accurately reflect all aspects of your agreement with the agency. I guarantee your agency takes them seriously . . . and you should too!*

Here's a couple of examples showing the power of the contract:

* During an assignment, a traveler noticed it was difficult to schedule time off. The permanent staff had, shall we say, "priority". The facility wanted the traveler to extend. Since she had already planned to travel out of town to visit her granddaughter on a particular three day weekend, her recruiter wrote the time off dates into the contract extension. Everyone signed the extension. Sure enough as the date approached,

the traveler mentioned her time off and the scheduler had problems. Rather than arguing, the traveler simply stated, "It's in my contract". The schedule was quietly changed, she saw her granddaughter as planned, and nothing else was mentioned about it.

* A traveler signed a contract and reported to work only to discover there was a $30 monthly charge for parking at the hospital. She had never encountered that before and did not think to ask the question during the telephone interview. She called her recruiter seeking to be reimbursed for the charge. The answer: "Sorry, it's not in the contract you signed".

> **Insight** *Any contract worth its salt will have a statement saying something like, "This contract constitutes the full and complete understanding and agreement between the two parties". If that doesn't scare you into being sure it's complete and accurate, nothing will!*

Contract Clauses

Every agency will have a standard contract form that consists of at least three parts: the standard fixed-wording clauses, edited clauses describing the particulars for the assignment, and a signature area.

Standard clauses. These deal primarily with the agency's policy and procedures. They are carefully worded and remain the same in every contract issued by the agency. They are revised only if legal issues are encountered with the wording or if policy changes occur. Here are some of the issues that may be addressed by standard clauses:

* Your employment data and any facility/JCAHO requirements must be completed prior to the assignment.

* Policy for rental cars such as not accepting additional insurance or upgrades.

* Meals and other charges are not to be charged to the room.

* The agency and facility may terminate or extend assignments.

* The policy if you are terminated due to misconduct or inadequate job performance.

* Responsibility to submit time sheets in a timely manner.

* Housing move-in and move-out procedures including any required signed forms.

* Policy for notifying the agency of your availability at the end of the assignment.

* Non-competition policy if you accept a permanent job at your assignment facility.

* Requirement to maintain confidentiality as to the terms of your contract.

* Requirement to sign the contract prior to reporting for the assignment.

* If your agency offers 24/7 emergency support, those details should be stated.

And any other policy statements your agency feels are important.

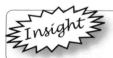 *I can assure you almost all of the standard clauses protect the agency, not you!*

Edited clauses. These paragraphs reflect the specific details of the assignment. They are in a fixed format for every contract but are edited to describe your duties and responsibilities, and the responsibilities of the facility and agency. By and large they protect you so be sure they are complete and accurate! They should include:

- The facility name, address, phone number.

- Point of contact, time to report on the first day, and attire for the first day.

- Starting and ending dates of the assignment.

- Requested days off and paid holidays during the assignment period.

- Hourly wage, length of the normal work day and work week, overtime rate and conditions for paying over-time. Shift differentials, weekend pay, call rate, and call back details. Rate of pay for holidays. Any other stipulations regarding wage-based pay.

- Daily per diem rate and details of other tax-free reim-bursements, such as travel allowance, car rental, etc.

- Any float requirements including units and estimated frequency.

- Applicable bonuses.

- Housing details should be included although they are sometimes provided in a separate document.

- A clause guaranteeing your hours.

And any other items you feel strongly about.

Signature area. There will be an area for you to sign and date, and an area for the agency representative (usually your recruiter) to sign and date.

In this age of word processing, contracts are not preprinted. As such they can easily be changed and printed as required. For legal reasons, your agency will almost certainly refuse to edit the standard clauses but there is no reason they cannot change the other portions of the contract if they do not accurately reflect the agreement and details of the assignment.

"Shall" and "Will"

Some formal contracts make extensive use of the terms "shall" and "will". They may seem interchangeable but the distinction is important to understand. "Shall" means the signer of the contract to do the work (you) must perform the action stated. "Will" means the action is to be performed by others, not you. As an example, here's the same sentence worded both ways:

> "All scrubs shall be provided."
> "All scrubs will be provided."

In the first sentence, you have to provide your own scrubs. In the second sentence the scrubs will be provided by someone else (probably the facility) and you do not need to provide them. Because of this inherent confusion with "shall" and "will", many contracts use expanded wording. Instead they may state something like:

> "The Healthcare Professional is responsible for providing their scrubs."

or

> "The Facility is responsible for providing scrubs to the Healthcare Professional."

Hopefully your agencies do not make extensive use of the "shall" and "will" wording. If they do, be sure to clarify any issues you do not fully understand.

Are Your Full Time Hours Guaranteed?

This is another subject that bears repeating. Your contract (or your agency's contract with the facility) should contain a provision guaranteeing full time employment per week. This keeps the facility from using you PRN and helps you receive the compensation you need and expect each pay period. In specialized areas, and perhaps even on the floors, the case load can vary significantly on a daily basis. The facility may also experience periods of low census. Some days you may work only several hours while other days may require overtime.

During those light work periods, your supervisor may "allow" you to leave early. Be careful about this. If you can leave and still get paid for it, great. Unfortunately, what they often mean is they will allow you to leave but not be paid for those hours off, and you may have to make up the hours later. And since your reimbursements for housing, daily living expenses, etc., are based on full employment each week, these items will be prorated and reduced as well. You really get the "double whamee" if you can't fill out your time sheet with at least your full time hours each week.

If you understand all this and still wish to take off during slack periods, fine. Also, if you have accumulated leave, you can use those hours to help fill in the gaps of your time sheet.

If your supervisor "allows" you to leave but you feel you need the hours, tell them exactly that: you need your full time hours per week to meet your obligations. If you have a guaranteed hours clause, they must allow you to stay, or pay you anyway. You may have to perform more routine tasks like restocking supplies, additional paper work such as policies and procedures, etc., but you can get your hours in. You may also have to float to other areas that need help. Such float must be within your abilities and fit under the general scope and intent of your contract. If you feel the facility is not using you as specified in your contract, call your recruiter. And this will be a great opportunity to see how well your agency stands up for you!

The Non-compete Clause

We breezed over this issue earlier when we were listing the fixed clauses of a contract. Occasionally a traveler under contract to an agency will decide to stop traveling and become a permanent staff member in that same job at that same facility. They simply convert to full time permanent status. Agencies may have a non-compete clause either in the contract with the traveler or with the facility. The stipulations vary but in general the traveler under contract to an agency can not accept a full time permanent position at that facility for six months to a year, (perhaps longer) after the assignment.

The agency may agree to release the traveler if a "head hunter" fee is paid to them by the facility.

Notes

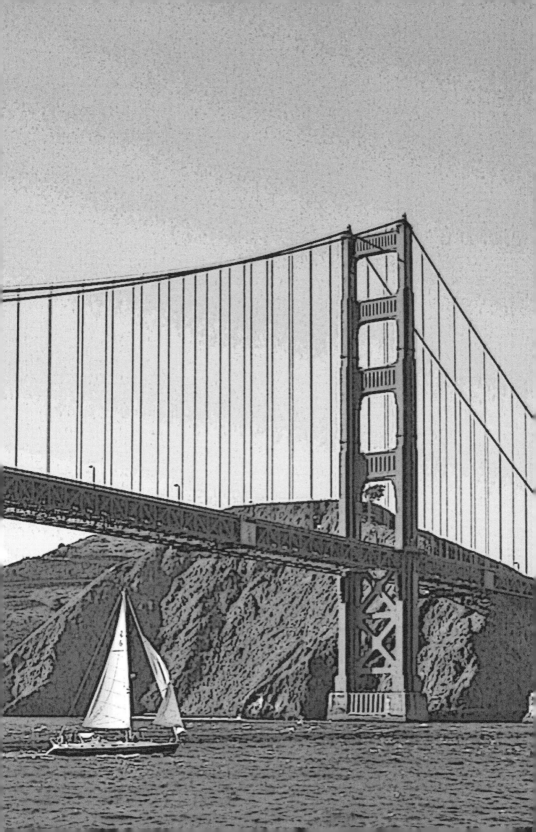

8

Your Compensation

*I could probably get along without money but my
credit card company is crazy about it.*

*A*s a traveler, you will likely make more per hour than at your old permanent job. In fact, there's a good chance you will make as much, or more, per hour as your permanent staff coworker doing the same job at the facility. Throw in housing at little or no cost to you, other tax-free money for living expenses, and it all adds up to quite a sum!

We have discussed a lot of important issues so far in Part Two: housing, benefits, tax advantage programs, taxes, and contracts. Now it's time to explore that topic near and dear to everyone. Of course I'm referring to your paycheck!

Again, compensation falls into two categories: taxable and non-taxable. Your personal situation will determine the tax status of some of your pay items. In this chapter we assume you meet the IRS criteria for tax-free reimbursement by maintaining a permanent home and accepting only temporary assignments that are far enough away from your home.

Taxable Compensation

We discussed the tax-free payment items Chapter 5. They include housing, daily living allowance, travel costs, etc. These items plus your taxable wages make up your total pay package. Here's a look at what's taxable:

Hourly wages. This is the base hourly wage you are paid.

Overtime. You should get at least time and a half for all overtime worked. A few assignments pay double time, but this is not the norm.

On call. The number of hours you carry a beeper multiplied by the hourly on call rate.

Call back. The number of hours actually called back while on call multiplied by your hourly call back rate. Some contracts specify a minimum number of hours paid for call back. For example, if you are called in but the case is canceled you may receive two hours of call back pay. Depending on when you are called in, a shift differential may also apply.

Bonuses. Any bonuses you receive should be taxable. This includes payment for such items as sign-on, completion, referral, loyalty, and extension.

Estimating Your Paycheck

Will you really make more money as a traveler? Time to put it to the test! Let's estimate some paychecks and you can be the judge. We'll use two examples and calculate the first and normal paychecks for each. Of course, we'll have to make some assumptions.

Example 1

> You are paid weekly
> 40 hour work week
> Corporate housing is provided as a separate item
> $28 per hour taxable wage
> No overtime, call, or call back is assumed
> Health insurance costs you $100 per week
> $45 per day living expenses (M&IE)
> $800 travel costs ($400 on the first and last paychecks)
> $85 reimbursement for license cost in that state
> Work 46 weeks per year (take off six)

Your deductions for federal and state taxes, medicare, etc. will vary depending on your tax bracket, but a conservative rule of thumb for estimating is to reduce your taxable wages by about 30%, making it 70% of the original figure.

In this example your housing is furnished as a separately paid item and will not appear on your paycheck. Your first paycheck would be:

Taxable portion:
Gross wages: 40 hours * $28   = $1120
Deduct for taxes, etc. $1120 * 0.70 =   784
Deduct for health insurance   =   100
              Total net taxable wages = **$684**

Tax-free portion:
M&IE: $45 * 7 days   = $315
Travel costs: $800 / 2   =   400
License reimbursement   =   85
              Total tax-free portion = **$800**

Total take home pay for your first check would be approximately $684 + $800 = **$1484.**

Without the one time payments of travel and license reimbursement, your normal weekly paycheck would be nearly **$1000** ($684 + $315).

Unless you work a lot of overtime, your first and last paychecks are usually the largest. They include your travel costs to and from the assignment and other one-time payments, such as any bonuses or license reimbursement.

Also notice your first paycheck had more tax-free reimbursement money than you made by working your shift ($800 vs. $784)!

So how much money would you make per year in our example? Assuming you work 46 weeks and take off six weeks during the year, you would make **$66,895**. Here's the breakdown:

Taxable weekly income is 46 weeks * $1120 = **$51,520**
Tax-free weekly income is 46 weeks * $315 =   **14,490**
Tax-free reimbursement for travel =   **800**
Tax-free license reimbursement =   **85**
                                           Total = **$66,895**

The **$51,520** would appear on your W-2 as taxable income and the remainder, about **$15,375** would be tax-free. In this example, **23%** of your yearly income ($15,375 / $66,895) would be tax-free.

And in our example, your housing is provided at no cost to you: paid as a separate item by the agency! You must still maintain your permanent home and pay all the bills associated with it, but you don't have to use any of your take home pay for rent or utilities for your assignment housing.

(*Example 2*)

Your agency may quote your assignment in terms of shifts. As an example let's say they offer:

Weekly pay
$550 total per shift
3 shifts per week, 12 hours each shift
Of the $550, $140 is a tax-free stipend (Lodging and M&IE)
No overtime, call, or call back is assumed
Health insurance costs you $100 per week
$800 travel costs ($400 on the first and last paychecks)
$85 reimbursement for license cost in that state
Work 46 weeks per year (take off six)

Given this criteria let's calculate your first paycheck:

Taxable portion:
Gross wages ($550-$140) * 3 shifts = $1230
Deduct for taxes, etc. $1230 * 0.70 =   861
Deduct for health insurance   =   100
Total net taxable wages = **$761**

Tax-free portion:
$140 * 3 shifts   = $420
$800 travel / 2   =   400
License reimbursement   =   85
Total tax-free portion = **$905**

Total take home pay for the first check would be:
$761 + $905 = **$1666.**

Without the one time payments of travel and license reimbursement, your normal weekly take home pay would be **$1181** ($761 + $420).

How much money would you make per year in our example? Assuming you work 46 weeks and take off six weeks during the year, you would make **$76,785**. Here's the breakdown:

Taxable weekly income is 46 weeks * $1230 = **$56,580**
Tax-free weekly income is 46 weeks * $420 =   **19,320**
Tax-free reimbursement for travel =   **800**
Tax-free license reimbursement =   **85**

$$\text{Total} = \$76,785$$

The **$56,580** would appear on your W-2 as taxable income and the remaining **$20,205** would be tax-free. In this example, about **26%** of your yearly income ($20,205 / $76,785) would be tax-free.

All things being equal which offer is better? In the second example you take home more money per normal week ($1181 vs. $1000) and more of it is tax-free ($420 vs. $315). So obviously the second example is the best offer, right?

Not necessarily. In the first example your housing is paid separately. No money comes out of your pocket for rent, utilities, deposits, telephone, TV cable, etc. In the second example the tax-free reimbursements include a housing stipend. While this is more money each week, you are responsible for locating and paying for all housing costs. The difference in total take home pay ($181 per week) may not cover your housing costs. Example 1 may be the best offer.

All of this is well and good but suppose you make more or less than the $28 in our examples. Now that you see how things fit together you can generate your own estimates for your special circumstances. Also, your agency can give you the approximate weekly take home pay based on your situation and the assignment details.

Prorated Items for Working Less than Full Time

We have mentioned this item, but it is worth discussing in more detail. There are a lot of benefits to traveling but paid time off during the contract is not one of them! Depending on the agency's benefit package, you will probably not receive much paid leave time during your first year, and probably not much after that, either.

Working less than your full time hours each pay period can be **very** costly. Be sure you understand your agency's policy regarding deductions to your pay for those hours of work you miss either through sickness or agreed upon time off.

Your housing, daily living allowance, special parking costs, and other reimbursements are based on you working full time each pay period. If you are sick or need to take time off for a short period, say a day or two, and do not have paid leave to cover it, not only will you lose the hourly pay for the hours missed, but the items mentioned may be pro-rated (reduced) as well. Also, if the total number of hours per contract period cannot be worked, a completion bonus may also be in jeopardy.

Here's an example of how expensive even a small amount of time off can be. Let's say your sister visited you for the weekend and needs to leave by plane on Monday morning. Between going to the airport and getting back, you will miss 5 hours of work that day. Let's also assume you work 8 hours per day, 40 hours per week, and receive the following pay items:
  $28/per hour wages
  $45/day M&IE
  $500 completion bonus
  $1700/month housing paid separately by your agency.

Here's what you lose:
Lost wages: $28/hr * 5 hrs = $140 * 0.70(taxes, etc.) = $98
Lost M&IE: $45/day * 7days * 5/40hours = $39
Housing cost you must reimbursed your agency:
[$1700/mo / (4.33 wks/mo * 40 hrs/wk)] * 5 hrs = $49

Total cost for missing 5 hours of work is almost **$186**.

Again, if you cannot make up the total contract hours, your completion bonus may be pro-rated or eliminated! A fairly expensive trip to the airport! Don't work less than your full time hours each pay period unless its absolutely necessary. It's simply too costly. Try to plan your off time before or after each assignment, or with permission of your supervisor, by adjusting the shift schedule.

A Word About Blended Rates

Some agencies quote a "blended" hourly rate. This is an average hourly wage often associated with 12 hour shifts. They pay a base rate for the first eight hours then the overtime rate for the last four. The total amount paid is then averaged for the twelve hours and this blended hourly rate is quoted to you. This is higher than the base rate and can be confusing.

As an example let's say your base rate is $28 per hour, your overtime rate is time and one half after 8 hours, and your shift is twelve hours. What is your blended rate?

Your eight hour shift pays $28 * 8 hrs   = $224
Your four hours O/T pays $28 * 4 * 1.5 hrs =   168
                                          Total = $392

The 12 hour shift pays a total of $392. When you divide it by 12 hours you get **$32.67** average per hour as a blended rate. You can see this blended rate is higher than the actual base hourly wage of **$28**.

Once you see how it goes you can use a general equation. If we let BHW equal the base hourly wage and BR equal the blended rate, the general equation for the example above is:

8*BHW + 4*BHW*1.5 = 12*BR   solving for BR leads to:
8*28 + 4*28*1.5 = 12*BR
[224 + 168] / 12 = BR
$32.67 = the Blended Rate

You can use the same relationship to determine your base hourly wage if the agency quotes a 12 hour blended rate. To check our first example let's now solve for the Base Hourly Wage (BHW):

8*BHW + 4*BHW*1.5 = 12*BR   solving for BHW leads to:
8*BHW + 4*BHW*1.5 = 12*32.67
BHW * [8 + (4*1.5)] = 392
BHW * 14 = 392
BHW = 392 / 14
Base Hourly Wage = **$28**

If you want to do the math you will find the relationships for our 12 hour example shift can be simplified to:

⚬ If you are given the Base Hourly Wage,
multiply it by 1.167 to find the Blended Rate.

⚬ If you are given the Blended Rate,
multiply it by 0.857 to find the Base Hourly Rate.

The bottom line is if an agency quotes an hourly rate for a shift over eight hours, be sure you understand if it's the base rate or a blended rate including overtime.

Verify Your Paycheck Accuracy

Your agency will make every effort to pay you accurately and on time but they also need your help. The time sheet is often a three part form so be sure to write legibly (and firmly) so that all copies can be easily read. The top copy (original) is for the agency, the other two copies are for you and the facility. Be sure it is filled out completely and that you and a representative of the facility sign the form.

The pay week usually runs from Monday through Sunday. Agencies will want to receive a faxed copy of the signed time sheet from the previous week as early on Monday morning as possible so they can process the payroll for that pay period. They also want to receive the original top copy by mail in a reasonable amount of time, normally within a week.

Insight *As a practical matter, we wait until we have three or four completed time sheets and then mail the originals to the agency in one envelope. While this may technically violate their policy, they seem to be OK with it. They already have the faxed copies to work from but ultimately need the originals to make their records complete.*

Input errors can occur so compare your time sheet to the pay stub for each pay period and report any discrepancies to your recruiter. They should correct the items on the next pay check.

And be sure you understand how the time sheet is to be filled out. One traveler had a strange experience along these lines. They noticed that sometimes when an odd hour figure such as 2 hours and 50 minutes was entered on the time sheet, it showed up as 2.5 hours on the pay stub. If the time was 4 hours and 30 minutes it appeared as 4.3 hours. This shorted the paycheck slightly for those hours. It didn't happen all the time, just occasionally. Apparently an office worker at the agency converted the hours to decimal before sending the time sheets to the payroll group. But occasionally this person was on leave and it did not get done, thus the errors. What this means is the payroll group could not (or would not) convert minutes to decimal of an hour to record the time correctly, and pay the traveler properly. To avoid this problem, the traveler began to convert the odd hours to decimal herself for the time sheet. After all, you don't want to make a bunch of "pencil pushers" work too hard!

If this becomes an issue for you, simply divide the minute portion by 60 and append it to the hour figure. As an example, for 9 hours and 48 minutes, divide 48 by 60 to get 0.80. Append it to 9 and it becomes 9.80 hours. The following chart may help. It shows minutes converted to decimal of an hour in five minute increments:

Convert Minutes to Decimal

Minutes	Divided by 60	Use
5	0.083	0.09
10	0.167	0.17
15	0.250	0.25
20	0.333	0.34
25	0.417	0.42
30	0.500	0.50
35	0.583	0.59
40	0.667	0.67
45	0.750	0.75
50	0.833	0.84
55	0.917	0.92

Thus 4 hours and 35 minutes equals 4.59 hours, and 2 hours and 20 minutes equals 2.34 hours. If you have to do this conversion for someone else's convenience, I would always round up as shown in column 3. It will not make much difference to your wallet but you'll feel better!

Holiday Pay

As a permanent staffer, you may have received at least time and one half for working holidays. As a traveler your contract should contain a list of holidays and the policy for receiving holiday pay. Most facilities (and agencies) require you to work the workday before and the workday after in order to receive overtime pay for a holiday. Be sure you understand the policy and the holiday pay rate. You don't want any surprises on your paycheck! Regardless of your agency's policy you still may not be paid overtime for working holidays. Why? The facility may simply revise your work schedule to avoid this payout.

Notes

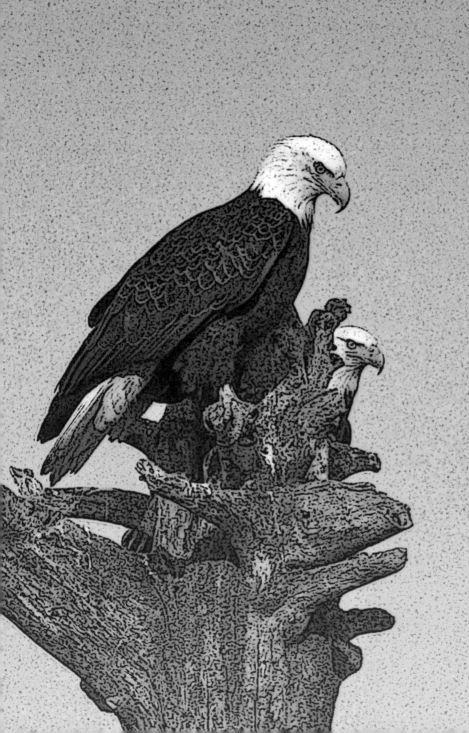

9

Licensing

*The way things are going you'll have to be
fingerprinted to pass through those Pearly Gates.*

*L*icensing can be expensive and time consuming. It pays to . . .

Plan Ahead

If you require a license to practice, you may wish to apply ahead of
time to at least those states you would like to visit. This helps prepare
you for that special assignment you want and increases your marketability. Your agencies can also provide a general idea where their
contracts are located and the areas where the greatest need for your
specialty may exist.

In this age of increased security, licensing can take longer than you
might expect. Fingerprinting and background checks are the norm.
The state may issue a temporary license quickly, but it's not unusual
to take 4-8 weeks (or longer) to get your permanent license. And the
FBI sometimes rejects fingerprint cards as unreadable, making you
re-submit them.

> ⚡**Insight**⚡ Many healthcare workers have weak fingerprint ridges due to the need to constantly wash their hands. Some use Cornhusker's Lotion to raise their fingerprint ridges prior to fingerprinting. The FBI uses a compound called "Ridge Builder" to enhance the fingerprint pattern.

If you are a new traveler and have a list of places you want to visit, consider applying for all the licenses at the same time. Some states require verifications of **all** your existing licenses. Let's say you are licensed only in Alabama but want licenses in ten other states. By applying to all ten states at the same time, you only have to verify the Alabama license. This can ultimately save you time and money.

Of course, most of the hassle of applying, verifying, and fingerprinting could be solved with a "national" licensing system. We are slowly moving toward that goal by way of the . . .

Nurse Licensure Compact

In 1996 the National Council of State Boards of Nursing (NCSBN) began investigating mutual recognition models. Such a system would allow member states to recognize each other's licenses and would facilitate employment across state lines.

In 1997 they endorsed a model and established the Nurse Licensure Compact Administrators (NLCA) to develop rules to implement and manage it. The RN and LPN/VN Compact began in January 2000 with Maryland, Texas, Utah, and Wisconsin. As of this writing, 23 states have adopted the compact and every year or so another state joins. Here is a list of the members and the year they joined, from the NCSBN web site www.ncsbn.org (January 2009).

Arizona	2002
Arkansas	2000

Colorado	2007
Delaware	2000
Idaho	2001
Iowa	2000
Kentucky	2007
Maine	2001
Maryland	2000
Mississippi	2001
Nebraska	2001
New Hampshire	2006
New Mexico	2004
North Carolina	2000
North Dakota	2004
Rhode Island	2008
South Carolina	2006
South Dakota	2001
Tennessee	2003
Texas	2000
Utah	2000
Virginia	2005
Wisconsin	2000

Remember the compact only applies to RN, LPN, and VN licenses. Each compact state designates a Nurse Licensure Compact Administrator (NLCA) to exchange information between the states to promote compliance. One of the data items shared is disciplinary action regarding the licensee.

Can you benefit from the compact? The answer is "yes" if you reside in and have a license in a member state. Your residency is defined as your permanent home for tax purposes.

The compact allows you to work in any other member state under your resident state license. When a state joins the compact they re-issue licenses to their residents identifying them as members of a compact state. Keep in mind you will have to abide by any state laws where you are practicing and you will have to be in good standing in your home state.

If your state of residency is not a member of the compact, there are no benefits to you. As far as you are concerned the compact does not exist. If you wish to practice in any state (compact or not), you will have to apply to that state for a license that can only be used in that state. Also, if you have a compact license and wish to work in a non-compact state, you will have to apply just as in "the good old days". Your compact license will not help in this instance.

The compact provides enormous benefits to those eligible. The licensee can work in member states under their resident license. No more fingerprinting, background checks, delays, and multiple license fees to be able to work across state lines.

Changing your permanent residence can impact your compact license, even if you move from one compact state to another. Both states should be notified. Your new resident state will issue a new compact license to you. Your former resident state will cancel your original license.

> *Insight* *Given the hassle of getting a license, the state police and FBI should insist that all states join the compact. It would greatly reduce their nightmare workload for fingerprinting and background checks.*

Walk-through States

Some states are known as "walk-through". This means you can generally get your temporary license the same day you arrive and apply at their office. As of this writing you can walk through:

California

Colorado

Delaware

District of Columbia

Idaho

Kansas

Maine

Maryland

Missouri

Nebraska

North Carolina

South Caroline

South Dakota

Vermont

Most states will grant a temporary license fairly quickly to allow you to start work. If time is tight and you are planning to get a license from a walk-though state, check ahead with the state board to be sure they still allow the walk-through process.

Insight *Even if you are applying to a walk-through state, call their office prior to arriving to see exactly what is required and the best way to verify your other licenses. The verification process is aided by those states using Nursys, although there is a cost to you for the service. Some states will accept verification via fax. Just be sure you understand what's involved to minimize potential delays, especially if time is tight for your assignment start date.*

License Renewal

Most states require license renewal every two years. A few renew yearly. Almost all states require continuing education units (CEU's) for renewal and some may specify certain required courses. By planning ahead you should be able to satisfy these requirements with local courses and seminars, perhaps through your facility at little or no cost. If you find yourself lacking CEU's for renewal, several online providers can help. Of course it will cost, but that's better than letting your license lapse or getting caught during an audit. The trend lately is to allow renewals online using a credit card. This makes things quick and easy. Be sure to print the screen receipt or at least write down the confirmation details in case problems develop later.

If you have to renew your license while on assignment, talk to your recruiter about reimbursing you for the cost.

Boards of Nursing

Rather than listing the individual Boards of Nursing here (the information is constantly changing), I suggest you bookmark the web site for the National Council of State Boards of Nursing (www.ncsbn.org). They have the latest information on the Nurse Licensure Compact and also maintain a current list of the Boards of Nursing for all the states, the District of Columbia, and the U.S. territories. The list includes their mailing address, fax and phone numbers, points of contact, and web site link.

Another notable site is www.allnursingschools.com. On their Articles & Resources page, Nursing Continuing Education link, they list the Board of Nursing information for the 50 states and the District of Columbia. They do not have a direct link to the web sites, nor do they have information pertaining to the U.S. territories. However, they include information on initial and renewal fees along with CEU requirements for each state, and the District of Columbia.

These and other web sites can be found by using a search string such as "Boards of Nursing". Of course, the individual site for a state board can be located by using its name in a search string such as "Alaska Board of Nursing".

Notes

Notes

Notes

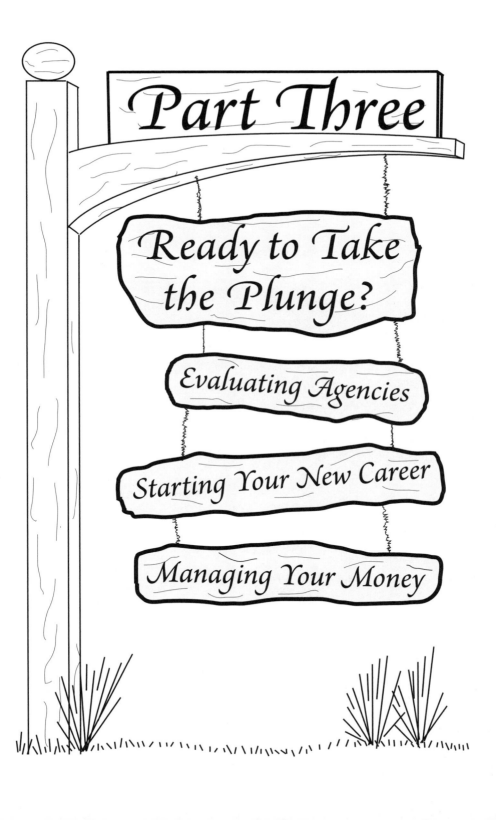

Part Three

Ready to Take the Plunge?

Evaluating Agencies

Starting Your New Career

Managing Your Money

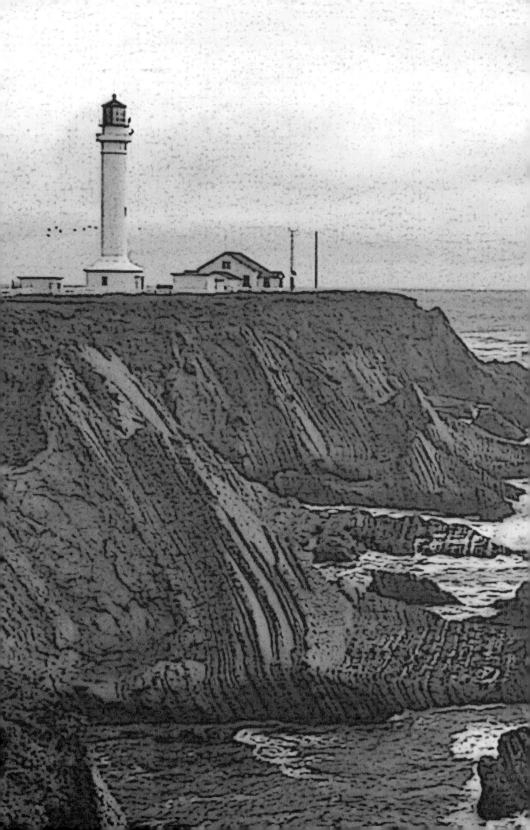

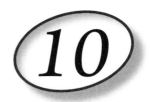

Evaluating Agencies

When discussing agencies I am quickly
reminded of one of my favorite movies:
"The Good, the Bad, and the Ugly".

Questions abound in the world of traveling but probably the most often asked is . . .

Which Agency Should I Choose?

One of the most important decisions a traveler makes is choosing one or more staffing agencies to work with. After all, unless you are an independent contractor, staffing agencies will place you in your assignments. You want agencies that will allow you to travel to the places you have always dreamed. You want good pay, good housing, benefits, and to be treated fairly. You also want them to be flexible when unexpected situations or costs are encountered. Of course you'll never really know how flexible your agency is until you have to face those situations. With well over 200 agencies in the U.S. to choose from, the task seems not just difficult, but almost impossible.

Agencies come in all sizes and flavors. Some are large and some are small. Some are local, national, or international. Some have been in business for many years and others have just arrived on the scene. Some offer comprehensive benefits. Others offer less, aiming to put more responsibility on the traveler but also more money in their pocket. Each agency will mix and match their housing options, benefits, assignment locations, and specialties they place. Many offer per diem work and permanent placement as well as opportunities for travelers. Here are some of the general categories and issues associated with agencies:

Local agencies. These focus on smaller areas such as New Orleans, Chicago, or San Diego. They place temporary workers for per diem registry work, permanent placement, and may have opportunities for travelers in that area as well. They generally offer a good hourly wage but fewer benefits.

Regional agencies. These focus on certain areas of the country such as the Northeast, the Southwest, or an individual state such as California, New York, or Pennsylvania. They, too, can have a mixture of offerings for per diem, permanent placement, and travelers.

Nationwide agencies. While these too can offer per diem and permanent placement, they often focus on opportunities for travelers. These agencies usually offer a broad range of assignments and locations with a full array of benefits and housing options. However, some agencies use the term "across the Nation" rather loosely. When interviewing them ask where most of their contracts are and what specialties they place.

International agencies. These agencies offer opportunities for foreign healthcare workers to live and work in the U.S. and provide opportunities for U.S. healthcare workers to be placed abroad.

Specialty agencies. These tend to place one or only a few specialties. Dialysis, physical therapists, and CRNA's come to mind. Per diem, permanent placement, and travel assignments are often available through these agencies.

Large verses small, old verses new. Each type has advantages and disadvantages. The larger agencies are often older and more established. You would expect them to have more contracts and thus more opportunities. However, larger size can indicate a certain bureaucratic "stiffness" and less personal contact. If they have enough travelers under contract they may become complacent about their business, choosing instead to "rest on their laurels".

Smaller or newer agencies may give exceptional personal service but may have a limited number of opportunities. However, they may be more aggressive in seeking new contracts to expand their business. As they grow, it becomes difficult to do everything at a personal level. And being certified by JCAHO adds a layer of rigidity to any business structure.

> *Insight*
>
> *A traveler's agency was fairly small when they started, but over the years the agency grew several fold. The traveler still gets good assignments, with good pay and service but some of the procedures are more formal. They often get a form letter now rather than a personal e-mail or phone call.*

Recruiters can make all the difference. You may get excellent service from a large agency and poor service from a smaller one depending on the personality and work ethic of your recruiter. So how do you choose agencies?

Decide what issues are important to you. Do you want top wages no matter where the assignment is located? Are you willing to sacrifice some in wages and benefits to work in certain areas of the country? Do you want only private housing? Do you want comprehensive health benefits, or are you willing to find your own medical coverage? Pick out three or four "show stoppers" as criteria to be used to weed out agencies. These are items you are reluctant to compromise.

Then pick out several "tie breakers". These are items that are important but are secondary and ultimately could be sacrificed if you really want a particular assignment. Your "tie breakers" will further help eliminate agencies. They may include such things as matching 401(k) funds, license reimbursement, life insurance, etc.

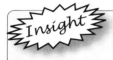 *Only you can decide what is important to you. Most travelers seem to be interested in pay rates, assignment locations, quality housing, and good medical benefits.*

Start your search for agencies. After you have determined your show stoppers and tie breakers, begin your search for agencies that fill the bill. Of course, the best way to learn of agencies is by word of mouth. If possible, talk to travelers about their experiences. Ask them to be candid. Perhaps they have dealt with several agencies and have one or two they prefer (and some they recommend avoiding).

In Chapter 2 we talked about some of the internet resources dealing with the issues of traveling. Tune into the discussion forums to see what other travelers are saying about different agencies. Post your own questions and search back several months for previous comments. You can also find valuable information by using search strings such as "travel nurse", "travel nursing", "traveling nurse", and "travel nursing jobs".

Almost every agency will have a web site describing their opportunities and the highlights of their benefit package. The web sites are important in that they stress what the agency would like you to know about them. But they never give all the details. Often they are most informative for what they omit. For instance if "furnished housing" is mentioned, it may be shared, not private. Otherwise it would have probably said "private furnished housing". If a 401(k) plan is offered but there is no mention of matching funds by the agency, guess what? They probably don't offer it.

Follow up with phone calls to the agencies you feel may meet your needs. Have a current resume ready to e-mail to them. This will give them an idea of your qualifications and experience. Ask about those specific issues that are most important, especially your show stoppers and tie breakers. You should be able to discover what is generally offered for most assignments, including the pay range for your specialty, tax advantage programs, medical insurance, etc. Some specialties are in more demand than others. Ask how easy or difficult it is to place travelers with your experience and specialty. Some agencies may have limited contracts in your area of expertise. For instance if you are a Cardiovascular Tech, you would probably want to sign with agencies that either specialize in, or at least have a significant number of cath lab contracts.

> *Insight* *If a traveler has suggested an agency, mention their name when you talk to the recruiter. If you ultimately accept and complete an assignment with that agency, the traveler should get a referral bonus.*

As mentioned earlier, you may not require some of the benefits offered. If so, ask if the equivalent value can be added to your pay package. If you want to travel with a pet, or use an RV, find out what's involved. Try to cover all the basic concerns that are important to you.

When interviewing agencies, their attitude toward you is just as important as the information they provide. How well do they listen? Do they ask questions about your situation and goals? Do they suggest possibilities that directly address **your** interest and not necessarily theirs? Do they seem interested in trying to get you to the places you desire? Or do they seem to want to steer you to certain locations (perhaps where they can make the most money or to the hard to fill assignments). You need to have a "warm, fuzzy" feeling about the agency and especially the recruiter. They need to assign you to locations you want to go, but just as important, to place you in situations where you best fit. Your gut feeling about a recruiter and an agency is probably the best. Trust your instincts!

If you accept an assignment and it doesn't work out for any reason, use that contract period to contact other agencies for your next assignment! Remember you are only obligated to that agency for the life of the contract you have signed.

> **Insight** *A few agencies want you to fill out an application and submit a lot of forms before they will even talk to you. Apparently, some recruiters earn money by simply adding applicants to their rolls. Tell them you are in the preliminary phase of selecting an agency and are seeking general information.*
>
> *If discussions progress and it looks like it may work out, there will be plenty of time to send the formal paperwork. Offer to e-mail a current resume to them. This will have enough information about your qualifications and experience for them to begin talking to you about traveling. I suggest moving on if the agency refuses to discuss issues with you until you have formally applied.*

Suggested Questions for Agencies

Focus on asking generalized questions when you first contact an agency. Remember you are weeding them out based on the "big picture" of what they offer and how they operate. If you wish to continue to talk to an agency there is plenty of time to ask about the "nitty gritty" details, especially when discussing a potential assignment. Here are a few general questions you might ask to help you eliminate some of the agencies:

* How long have you been in business?
* How many recruiters do you have?
* What specialties do you place?
* What areas of the country are your contracts located?
* Do you have many contracts for my specialty?
* Can you give me a "ballpark" range for my hourly wage?

* Are my hours guaranteed?
* What housing options do you offer?
* Is it OK to travel with a pet?
* Do you offer medical benefits? What are the options? How are pre-existing conditions handled?
* Do you offer a 401(k)? Is it matched? Is there a waiting period to join? How soon will I be vested?
* Do you offer a tax advantaged program? How are the items allocated? (Per hour basis or separated by item)
* What other benefits are offered?
* If I don't need a particular benefit, can I receive the equivalent amount as a pay increase?
* How does travel to and from assignments work? If I fly will you pay for a rental car?

And any other general questions you feel are appropriate.

The Application Process

When you have narrowed your choice to several agencies (perhaps five at most), consider applying to all of them. By now you should have a good feeling about your potential recruiters. They should have indicated a narrow range of pay you can expect for your specialty and at least a rough idea of potential assignments. You should understand their benefits package, what to expect in your housing, and what tax-free reimbursements you will receive. Of course the exact dollar amounts will change for each assignment, but there should be no big surprises left to encounter.

The requirements to sign-up with an agency can vary but these are generally required:

* At least one year of recent verifiable experience in the specialty you plan to work

※ Pass online tests as required
※ Have clinically-based employment references
※ Evidence of good health including a recent physical examination. TB screening, Rubella, Rubeola, Mumps, and Varicella immunity
※ BCLS certification ACLS/NRP/PALS as applicable
※ A current license (if required) in the state you are now working

You will also have to submit several forms to the agency including:

※ Application form
※ Direct deposit form
※ W-4 IRS withholding form for payroll
※ I-9 INS form to prove eligibility to work in the U.S.
※ Permanent tax home declaration form
※ Health form to document physical exam and immunizations
※ Hepatitis declination form
※ HIPAA form
※ OSHA orientation checklist
※ Skills checklist

The agency will prefer to have all required forms on file so you are ready to go quickly when an assignment becomes available. A few of the forms, such as your direct deposit and W-4 withholding, contain sensitive information. You may wish to submit those only after it looks like you will be accepting an assignment. They can be sent to the agency quickly, and have no effect on your qualifications for employment.

Once you have formally applied to your agencies and given them a tentative start date they can begin a serious search for an assignment and will be more specific about the openings available. Remember, applying to an agency in no way obligates you to work for them. You will merely be in their system as a potential traveler.

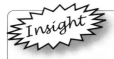 *Some agencies run a credit check on their applicants. Ask your recruiters if they have this policy and "opt out" if you feel uncomfortable for any reason.*

JCAHO Certification

The Joint Commission on Accreditation of Healthcare Organizations (JCAHO) has set standards for staffing agencies. JCAHO certification is not often required but staffing agencies are finding it easier to place travelers if they are certified. It gives the facilities an added level of confidence when dealing with an agency. Of course, this means more work (and cost) for the agency and more paperwork for their travelers.

The JCAHO-certified agency is required to adhere to certain organizational structure. They are expected to establish formal job duties and positions for such things as payroll, housing, benefits, quality assurance, administration, etc. Most staffing agencies have at least the bare bones structure in place to conduct business, but JCAHO forces a more rigid, organized business model with defined duties. The certification also mandates certain fair business practices and ethical conduct. A formal complaint procedure is in place for those that have issues. This certification comes at a price. JCAHO charges a fee for this service and the agency must keep their documentation current and renew their certification every two years.

As a traveler you will also feel the burden of JCAHO if your agency is certified. They will need certain documentation from you for their files. Periodically submitting copies of your credentials and passing online tests are the norm. Don't be too upset with the QA person. Their job is to be sure all documentation is in place. And travelers are notorious for dragging their feet on this issue. Do your best to work with them. JCAHO certification ultimately benefits all concerned.

> **Insight** *Some individual facilities and hospital associations are now requiring staffing agencies to be certified by JCAHO. If you feel JCAHO certification is important, you may wish to use it as one of your criteria when evaluating agencies.*

Agency Listings on the Internet

Originally I planned to provide a listing of agencies for reference. However I quickly discovered the "landscape" is constantly changing and any printed list would quickly be out of date. While many agencies are well established, others come and go: sometimes rather quickly. New agencies are popping up all the time. Some merge, some are bought out by others, and some simply go out of business.

I suggest using the internet to get as current a list of agencies as possible. As mentioned in the Internet Resources section of Chapter Two, www.travelnursetoolbox.com does a good job of maintaining a list of agencies and provides a link to each agency's web site.

And of course, search strings such as "travel nurse agencies" or "travel nurse jobs" may provide additional information.

Notes

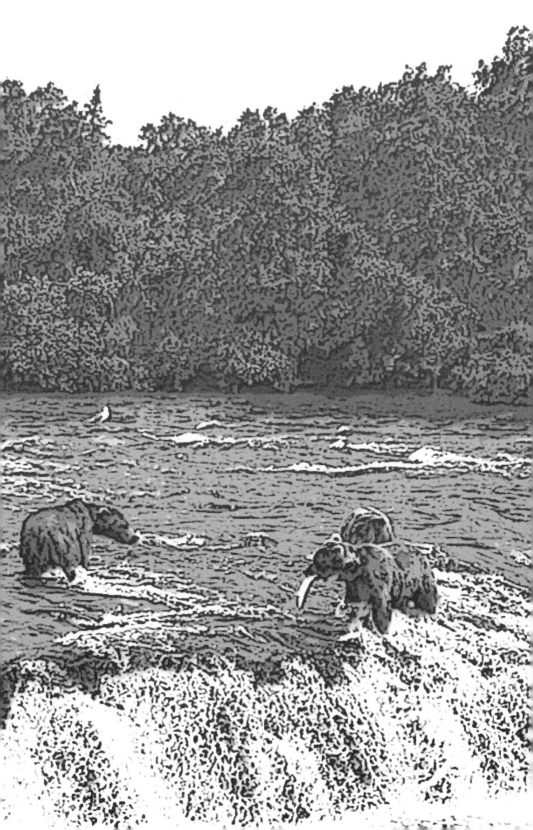

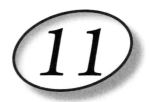

Starting Your New Career

What's that sound I hear?
Is it Opportunity knocking?

Well, you're at that point! Are you ready to take the giant leap? Is traveling right for you? If it is, have you chosen a few agencies you think will work with you? Are they optimistic about getting you an assignment you will like? Do you think you're ready for a change in lifestyle? Do you feel good about your decision? If so it's time to think about . . .

Getting That First Assignment

The transition from your old job to your first assignment can be somewhat of a balancing act. You don't want to resign, convert to PRN, or take a leave of absence until you have at least some assurance of a travel assignment. But given the fact that assignments can open and close quickly, your agencies can't seriously talk about specific assignments until you give them a tentative start date. How do you proceed? You have to juggle the two. Things can move slowly or very quickly!

> *Don't change your permanent job status until you have saved enough money to meet your expenditures during your transition, and feel good about an assignment from one or more agencies. Be realistic about your financial needs. There's not much worse than leaving a job, being in limbo, and watching your savings melt away.*

When your savings are in place, notify your agencies of a tentative start date. This is your best guess as to the first day it is possible for you to begin work at a travel assignment. The date is not chiseled in stone, but a reasonably close estimate as to your true availability. Keep in mind you will need to give sufficient notice before leaving your permanent job, prepare your home prior to leaving, take care of last minute items, and travel to the assignment. Be sure to give yourself some leeway.

Using this availability date, your agencies will begin searching for possible assignments. They may have something for you to consider immediately or it could take several days or perhaps a week or more. But don't panic. You still have your permanent job. If nothing happens right away you can just keep working. Check with your recruiters every several days if you have not heard from them. The agencies will work hard to find an assignment. After all, they make money by filling assignments!

When a recruiter has an assignment they will call you with the details. This should include location, length of the contract, pay rate, the hours per shift and per week, call, float required, etc. They may also know other items such as patient ratio, if scrubs are provided and any special fee for parking. Given your tax status, they should be able to estimate your take home pay each pay period. Also, they should have a good idea of available housing, especially if they have placed travelers at the facility before. You will have enough information to decide if you wish to pursue the assignment. They may have only one assignment or several for you to consider. Exactly when to change your job status is a judgment call based on how soon you feel your agencies can place you.

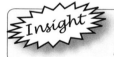 *The best situation is for your recruiters to come up with possible assignments during your permanent job notice period.*

If one or more assignments sound interesting, you are ready to "talk turkey".

Negotiating Your First Contract

The agency will work hard to place you. They want to demonstrate they can find assignments to your liking . . . and they want to start receiving the income your assignment generates!

Even so when they call you with an assignment their initial negotiating attitude, while friendly and polite, will be, "Here's the job. It pays this much. We'll send you the contract." They are attempting to gain the upper hand by having you assume they are holding all the cards.

And let's face it, for your first assignment they are in a strong negotiating position. As an unproven commodity to the agency (and to traveling in general), your negotiating clout for your first assignment will be minimal. It may be difficult to negotiate seriously until you have some traveling experience and they are convinced you are valuable. But this does not necessarily mean they will try to take advantage of you. If they can give you a good deal, place you successfully, and you have a good experience, you may extend your contract and continue to work for the agency on future assignments. If it's a bad experience they may never see you (or the income you generate) again! But should you take their first offer as presented? Not necessarily.

Remember everything is negotiable. And I mean everything! Even down to the color and size of the rental car. Hopefully you will dwell on more important issues such as pay, housing, benefits, and tax-free reimbursements. However, if a small issue is important, make it a negotiation item. By now you should know a fairly narrow wage range you can expect. You can check the Government per diem tables to get an idea of the allowable tax-free reimbursements. Question the "numbers" for the assignment if you feel any are too low.

> **Insight** *Frankly, for your first assignment, if the numbers look good and you feel you will like the situation and location, I suggest you take it. Use it as a learning experience for future assignments. Later, as a seasoned traveler, you will have more experience in how things actually work "out there" and will be in a better negotiating position.*

If your recruiters have several assignments that seem acceptable, let them present you to all of them. They will fax your profile to the facilities for review. If the facility likes your qualifications, they will call the recruiter who then arranges a convenient time for you and the facility to have a telephone interview.

Keep in mind that any facility offering you an assignment will no doubt want you to start as soon as you can. They need the help! Be sure your recruiter explains your situation to them: you are a first time traveler in transition from your permanent job. Most facilities can wait two or three weeks if they feel they are getting a good worker. They will "huff and puff" and act like they can't . . . but they can.

The Telephone Interview

This is usually your first direct communication with the facility. It is normally a one-on-one with your potential supervisor, although several facility staffers may participate via a conference call. Your recruiter is usually not involved in the interview. This is your chance to get to know more about the facility, staff, and working conditions. It is also an opportunity for the facility to learn more about specific aspects of your experience that pertain to the assignment. And of course both you and they will attempt to gauge the personality and temperament of the other. Keep in mind the facility may be interviewing several candidates for the assignment.

The telephone interview deals with the actual working conditions and related items. It does not deal with any wage or benefit issues. Those are between you and your agency. ***Verify all the stipulations of employment to be sure your agency correctly understood the needs of the facility.*** Ask any questions you feel could be points of contention later, such as the start date, patient ratios, how much overtime is normally encountered, required float, to what areas, and how often, cost of parking, guaranteed hours per week, who provides scrubs, orientation details, etc. Ask if you are required to take any pre-employment tests such as the PBDS or BKAT, and find out the consequences if you do not pass. Also, be sure to mention any time off you require during the contract and any other personal circumstances that may affect the assignment. No item is too small. If it's important to you . . . ask!

Sometimes the interview is conducted by a Human Resources representative for the facility. While this is helpful, they may not know all the nuances associated with the day-in-day-out workload. If you feel you need more specific information to help you make a decision, arrange to talk to the unit manager prior to accepting. After all, you need to be sure the assignment is right for you!

As with any interview, professionalism and courtesy are expected. It is best to have a list of questions and concerns prior to the interview. Answer questions directly and truthfully. Be pleasant but not overly chatty.

Don't be too concerned if the facility does not call at the appointed time. It may not have anything to do with you. A sudden meeting or crises may have arisen. On rare occasions an existing traveler scheduled to leave may be reconsidering, or the facility may be reconsidering (once again) their decision to hire a traveler. In any event your recruiter needs to stress there is a limit to your patience. If you do not receive at least a courtesy call from the facility in 2-3 days, it's time to consider another assignment.

> **Insight** — *Even if the facility says they want you for the assignment, don't commit during the telephone interview. Simply end the conversation with the understanding that they should contact your recruiter with their final decision. When your recruiter calls, you have another chance to see if your agency can sweeten the pot.*

Finalizing the Assignment

If the facility wants you for the assignment, they will call your recruiter who then lets you know. You are now in a little better negotiating position. After all you have a facility who wants you for an assignment and the agency can almost smell that money coming in. Your agency may be willing to sweeten the deal if they think it will help finalize it. Remember the contract you sign is between you and the agency. The facility is not involved.

So when have you made a commitment to take the assignment? Most agencies feel if you have verbally accepted the assignment from the facility and/or your recruiter you have made a professional commitment to accept the assignment. So be sure you are satisfied with the terms of the assignment before committing either verbally or in writing.

After you and the agency agree on terms your recruiter will prepare the contract. They will sign in their signature block and send it to you for your signature. Often they overnight it. Examine the contract carefully. It should contain all the particulars as discussed. If not, don't be shy about making them change it and send you the corrected version. Some agencies e-mail or fax a preliminary copy for your review prior to mailing the official copy. This can head off potential wording problems and ultimately save time. They should send several items with the contract including blank time sheets, housing information, a map showing how to get to the facility, etc. Prior to starting each assignment you must pass a drug test. Your agency should include the required form (prepaid by them) in your contract package.

Once you are satisfied with the contract and the other details of the assignment, sign and return (not necessarily overnight) the contract and the other required forms. Many agencies will not sign a housing lease for you until they receive your signed contract.

And when the deal is signed, sealed, and delivered start packing for your first travel assignment!

Preparing To Leave Home

Wow, you finally did it! Are you excited? Nervous? Worried? A little scared? All of the above? Don't worry, we and every other traveler have shared those feelings. After all, you are about to embark on a whole new phase of your life!

Now it's time to get serious about leaving your home and hitting the road. Here are some things to consider:

What to pack. One of the hassles of being a traveler is the limited space when moving. Unless you are planning to drive a semi-truck, you will have to be selective on what you take, especially if you fly between assignments. Even RV's have limited space.

Be realistic about the clothes you need. Take enough to avoid having to wash too frequently but not so many to require a lot of space. Do you really need three sweaters and seven pairs of shoes? Call the housing manager and check the laundry situation. Is it in your apartment, on the premises, or across town? Plan the amount of clothing accordingly. The climate and time of year will also dictate certain clothing. Keep in mind if you decide to extend your contract or move directly to another assignment you may find yourself on the road during a different season of the year.

Even if you will have a fully furnished corporate apartment you may still want to take a few of your favorite kitchen items. A wine opener and a garlic press are a couple of the items sometimes lacking from the kitchen package. Some take their answer phone, their favorite clock radio, pictures of their family, and other personal items.

Depending on your housing package you may have to pack even more items. Some travelers take silverware, pots and pans, china, and even a TV and some furniture.

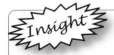 *The bottom line is: take only the items you really need. Other items can be purchased after you arrive.*

Your vehicle. If you plan to drive to your assignment be sure your vehicle is road worthy. Have a qualified mechanic inspect and test drive it if you don't feel comfortable doing so.

Here are some of the things to consider. Any hoses or belts that show cracks or weakness should be replaced. New tires are required if they are excessively worn or have developed a serious wear pattern. Does your car pull to one side? If so the front end may need aligning. Be sure your headlights, taillights, stop lights, and turn signals are working properly. If you can't remember when you last changed your oil and antifreeze, have them changed. If your battery is more than three years old consider changing it, especially if you are going to a cold weather region. If your car is older, consider changing the transmission and differential fluids. Be sure all fluids are at the proper level. Spark plugs, air cleaner, and fuel filter are other items of concern. Be sure your brakes and exhaust system are in good shape and that your heater and air conditioning function properly. Other items specific to your car also need checking, such as CV joints, all wheel drive, and four wheel drive components. If your car is "beyond hope", consider buying a different one. No one likes car payments or paying for car repairs. But it beats the risk of being stranded on the side of the road.

Be sure to carry a recent road atlas and consider a membership in a roadside assistance program in case you need help while traveling. Your car insurance company and car dealership may offer a plan. Other companies such as the American Automobile Association (AAA) offer the service. Check out the cost and options available. Some cars have built-in GPS as a navigational aid or you may wish to purchase a portable GPS unit.

Securing your home. If you are renting a house, apartment, or condo, you will probably want to continue renting it while on assignment. After all you need a place to call home: to rest and to work locally. You also need a permanent home for tax purposes. Let the rental manager know you are leaving so they can check periodically to be sure things are alright. Give them the assignment address and your phone number in case anything happens while you're away. Also, consider asking a trusted neighbor or family member to check on it periodically. You may want to leave one or more lights on timers to give the impression someone is still there.

If you are buying or own your own home, leaving is more involved. Hopefully a neighbor or family member can periodically check on it for you. Consider having an alarm system installed that is monitored. If the alarm goes off the monitoring service calls the police to respond. You will also need to arrange for normal maintenance is-sues such as lawn mowing, periodic inspection for your termite bond, house washing, etc.

Try to give your home a lived-in look while you are away. You can place lights on timers to simulate your normal activities while at home. We have our outside lights on dusk to daylight wall timers. If you leave a car in the driveway ask a neighbor to brush it off periodi-cally so it looks like it has been driven recently. Ask if they will start it occasionally to keep the battery charged. We set our thermostats at 78 for the summer and 60 for the winter. This keeps the house within reasonable temperature limits and saves on utilities.

> **Insight** *During our first assignment a toilet began to leak at our home. Fortunately a relative discovered it when checking the house. While it was a slow leak, if it had not been cor-rected it would have ruined the carpet throughout the house during our time away. We now turn the water off at the street prior to leaving.*

Last minute checklist. A final checklist can help prevent forgetting last minute items and procedures. As an example, here is the check-list we use:

- Unplug electronics.
- Put lights on timers.
- Take the telephone and clock radio.
- Turn hot water heater to "vacation".
- Flush toilets to put fresh water in the bowls.
- Set air conditioning/heating to proper settings.
- Take dog food, dog dishes, and leashes.
- Empty the trash.
- Turn water off at the street.
- Be sure all windows and doors are closed and locked.
- Turn off garage door opener.
- Set the house alarm.
- Lock the back door.

Surviving Your First Assignment

We talked about the need for sufficient savings prior to beginning your new career. You will also need a savings cushion at the start of every assignment. Please have access to enough money to meet all your needs for at least the first month (hopefully more).

Yeah . . . I know! You've been promised a furnished apartment, perhaps a rental car, daily living allowance for each and every day, travel costs, and no doubt a decent hourly wage. While the apartment, rental car and plane ticket (if flying) should be set up and pre-paid by your agency, you will not receive any cash (you know, that green stuff you put in your wallet) until the end of your second week of work if you are paid weekly, and probably not for a month if you are paid every two weeks. Until then you will need to cover expenses such as:

- Travel costs (gas, motels, etc.) if you drive a vehicle
- Your obligations for your new housing (if any)
- Food and incidentals
- Prescriptions
- Local parking and other transportation costs
- Entertainment
- Car payment and car costs such as insurance
- Other loan payments and credit card bills
- All bills associated with your permanent home

You should estimate your needs for this period and be sure you can access enough money while awaiting your first paycheck.

Coordinate with your agency and plan to arrive at least two days prior to the assignment. This will give you time to check-in, find the facility, and rest a little before starting work. Call your apartment manager at the assignment location prior to leaving home. Be sure the accommodations are as specified, and that they know to expect you. Try to avoid arriving on Sunday or very late on Saturday. Apartments sometimes work with limited staff then and those on duty may not have been told you are arriving.

> **Insight** It takes two or three weeks to feel comfortable at a new location. Finding your way around, including the closest and best food stores, restaurants, ATM's, pharmacies, banks, gas stations, etc., takes more time than you may think! Ask your coworkers for suggestions and buy a map of the local area.

Your first few days on assignment will be similar to starting any new job with one exception: you are expected to be fully competent when you walk through the door. Your orientation can be anywhere from a few hours to a week or more. But generally you are expected to have the knowledge and experience to hit the ground running.

Some permanent staff may be interested in the details of traveling, especially how much you make. They may have heard stories of travelers making huge sums of money. These are most often based on bill rates that have become public knowledge. They may think this is your hourly rate, and can sometimes cause resentment. Keep in mind you have signed a confidential agreement with your agency. If you are asked how much you make, simply brush it off as best you can. One good answer might be, "Just barely enough to pay my bills."

As work progresses remember what it takes to be a good traveler from Chapter 2. You are there to augment the permanent staff. Try to avoid turf issues and local politics. Learn their procedures, be friendly to all, and make suggestions tactfully.

Toward the end of your first contract re-evaluate everything. Has your agency performed as expected? Were you paid accurately and on time? Did they stand by you if difficult situations occurred? Did the facility and staff treat you well? Was the workload as expected? Did you have fun? Do you like traveling? Are you willing to extend if the facility asks, or is it time to move on?

Negotiating Your Contract Extension

If you fit in well, the facility may ask you to extend. After all, they probably still need help! Agencies expect you to extend under the same stipulations as the original contract. But keep in mind the extension is a separate and distinct contract. Everything is negotiable. Some travelers use this as a chance to ask for a little more. And your agency may be willing to go along with it. They already have you in place. They would have to find another traveler to fill the assignment and risk having it filled by a competitor. Can the agency bump up your hourly wage a little? Can they work on that per diem rate? Is a bonus possible?

Contract extensions are usually for 13 weeks just as the original contract, but they can cover more or less time. It may be getting close to the holidays and you only want to work a few more weeks, or the facility may be hiring a permanent staffer and wants you to fill in until they can get up to speed. Occasionally a facility may want you to extend for more than 13 weeks, say six months or longer. If you feel this meets your needs then fine, but many travelers enjoy the flexibility of shorter assignments in case that "dream" assignment suddenly opens.

Insight — *A traveler ended an assignment in mid-October and planned to take off until mid-January. Before she left, the facility asked her to sign a contract to return sometime after the New Year. She tactfully declined. She didn't want to obligate herself that far in advance. Who knows what opportunities can surface in three months?*

Subsequent Assignments

As we have seen, you can't predict exactly when openings will occur. They are very fluid. Facilities are constantly changing their needs. Personnel at the facility in charge of travel contracts are notorious for waiting until the last minute to commit. Also, the existing travelers at a facility can decide to extend at the last minute or the facility may be able to hire permanent staff to reduce the need for travelers. An opening this week at a particular location may not exist next week. An opening may suddenly exist at a facility that has never before used travelers.

Given this uncertainty, there is not much need in discussing future assignments until you are within the last month of your current assignment. At that time the facility should have a good idea if they want you to extend, and your agencies should have a better idea of what will be available if you wish to move on. We have a standing joke with our recruiters when we discuss new assignments. We ask, "Well what's on the radar screen ***this week***?"

This process can bother some, but it can be one of the exciting aspects of traveling. There is a sense of adventure in never really knowing where you are going until the last minute. You have to be patient, flexible . . . and prepared for almost anything. And every new assignment is a chance to try out your negotiating skills.

Insight

Even if you plan to extend your current contract, check with your agencies prior to signing. Who knows, that dream assignment you can't pass up may be opening at just the right time!

Negotiating Subsequent Contracts

If your first assignment goes well you will be in a better position to negotiate future assignments. Your agency now knows you are a valuable commodity. Even if you change agencies your new recruiter will appreciate the fact that you have traveled before. You no doubt have learned a lot from your first assignment. Apply your increased knowledge to your next contract negotiation. Here are a few tips that bear repeating:

Negotiate from strength. This is where a little financial stability helps. If your recruiters know you can ride out at least short term periods of unemployment, they may be more apt to pump the numbers up for an assignment they want to fill. The sooner they fill it, the sooner they start making money.

> **Insight** *We often take off for two to three months at the end of the year to be with family and friends during the Holidays. Recruiters sometimes call us up and ask, " Are you sure you don't want to go back to work now?"*

Don't appear overly eager. Every recruiter will ask which areas of the country you prefer and will try to get you there. However, they may be tempted to offer a lower package at first hoping you will accept. It is best to let your agencies know that even though you have preferences, you are open to other assignments. If a preferred assignment opens, be a little coy with the agency and try to get the best package you can. There will be plenty of time for your official "happy feet dance".

Keep in mind everyone needs to win. There is a limit to the negotiating flexibility of an agency. It is normally tied to the agency's budget for that assignment, which is tied to the bill rate. Everyone needs to benefit from the contract. And speaking of the bill rate . . .

Slicing Up the Bill Rate Pie

Let's take a moment to revisit this topic. As mentioned, the agency is paid the "bill rate" by the facility for every regular hour the traveler works. There are also stipulations for overtime, shift differentials, etc. Hourly bill rates may run between $55 and $78 or more depending on location and specialty. It is sliced into several portions. Some for you and a portion for the agency. Your portion provides wages, tax-free reimbursements, and most likely some benefits. The agency's portion pays for their salaries, operational costs, and includes their profit.

Maximizing your slice of the pie is difficult and you never really know how much money, if any, you left on the table. The problem is that some of the variables will be unknown to you. The agency will almost certainly not reveal their profit margin and will probably not reveal the assignment bill rate, although some do. Some may even be secretive about the total cost of housing. To show how the bill rate is generally sliced up, here's an example from one of our assignments. I made some assumptions as to the actual bill rate, the cost of housing, and agency profit. But they are close enough for our example. The agency furnished housing, paid a separate car allowance, and M&IE living expenses. Here's how the bill rate was apportioned:

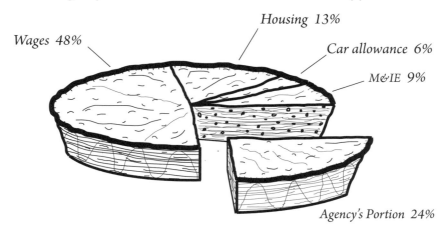

Wages 48%

Housing 13%

Car allowance 6%

M&IE 9%

Agency's Portion 24%

Assuming the same numbers, if we had received a stipend for housing and the car allowance had not been separated out from the M&IE, the pie would have looked like this:

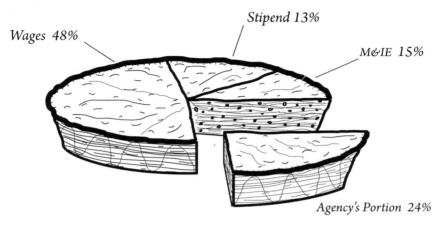

Stipend 13%

Wages 48%

M&IE 15%

Agency's Portion 24%

Your agency may pay you a housing stipend and your M&IE rolled into one daily per diem figure. Our example pie would then look like this:

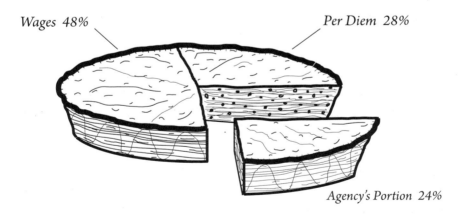

Wages 48%

Per Diem 28%

Agency's Portion 24%

Notice the amount paid for wages, housing, and tax-free reimbursements was the largest portion of the pie. Of the total, we received about 76% and wages made up nearly half the bill rate. Also, I did not include smaller reimbursements such as travel to and from the assignment, and license reimbursement. This would have increased our portion slightly.

Of course the actual percentages and dollar figures will vary for each assignment, and keep in mind the bill rate "pie" is only so big. If you expect more in wages, other portions of the pie adjust accordingly. And you can almost bet the agency's profit will not be one of those items adjusted! If you want more tax-free money, you may have to accept a slightly lower wage. Housing costs can vary dramatically and can have a large impact on your other slices.

> **Insight** — *Housing quality is often a sticking point with travelers. Your recruiter may say, "We are having trouble finding housing within the budget." One answer might be, "Reduce your profit a little and add it to the housing budget so I can live in something decent!"*

Actually, the agency may be willing to reduce the profit on an assignment if it will sweeten the pot and seal the deal. This is especially true if the agency has a long term traveler of proven quality, or if the assignment is hard to fill. No agency wants to lose a placement or a valued traveler over a few bucks per month.

Since you will be receiving the lion's share of the bill rate, shouldn't you be happy with the initial proposal from the agency? Well, maybe . . . and maybe not. Can that hourly wage be bumped up a little? How about that per diem rate?

In all phases of negotiations you must remain cordial, polite, and professional. Shouting and a belligerent attitude have no place. If you feel you have reached a temporary impasse, politely end the conversation by suggesting you need to think about it. Agree on a time to continue discussions. This pause can be beneficial to both parties. Each can think about what is really important. Do you really need license reimbursement to make this deal go? The agency may decide they are not willing to lose a placement over a dollar per hour.

At the end, both you and your agency need to feel the agreement is fair. Does this mean either is completely satisfied? Probably not, but it's a deal you both can live with.

Your Last Couple of Weeks on Assignment

Whether you are moving to another assignment or taking some time off there are several last minute items that need your attention prior to leaving.

Housing issues. Check with your local housing manager to see what date they have you leaving. You will often need a day or two after your assignment ends to finish packing and leave. Be sure your agency has rented the housing for the required extra time and that all utilities will still be active. If you are flying, check your ticket for the correct flight, time, and date.

> ***Insight*** *A traveler learned this housing lesson the hard way. The last day of a contract, and after the traveler had gone to work, their spouse discovered the TV cable and modem service had been disconnected, and that the furniture, etc., was going to be picked up around noon. The agency knew the traveler had to work a full shift that day and still needed to pack to leave the next morning. The agency had mistakenly set the utility cutoff and furnishings package pick-up date for the same date as the end of the contract. The spouse called the agency and they were able to correct everything in time. But if they had not been there, the traveler would have returned after work and found no furniture, no linens, no kitchen utensils, no TV or phone. Even the power may have been turned off.*

If you are responsible for utilities, telephone, TV cable, etc. notify those companies of the date to end service. Be sure they have your correct address to return any deposits. Make arrangements to have special equipment such as a cable modem picked up a day or two prior to leaving. More than one cable modem has "disappeared" after a traveler left and before the cable company arrived to pick it up.

If your agency provided your housing, they may require you to per-form a last minute walk through with a housing representative. The agency will often require a form be signed stating any items that are missing or damaged. This is for your protection and the agency's. It helps assure any deposits will be returned in a timely manner.

It's common courtesy to make a good faith effort to clean your hous-ing prior to leaving.

Food planning. Plan your meals and supplies more carefully during the last couple of weeks to avoid excess food and other items such as paper towels, soap, and toilet paper. Excess non-perishables can be donated to the local food bank.

Packing to leave. Double check all drawers, closets, and storage ar-eas to be sure you have all your items. If you brought personal items such as for the kitchen, be sure to pack only your items.

Last minute details. Bring your bills up to date and have enough cash to travel. Check to see if any prescriptions need refilling. If driv-ing, be sure your vehicle is road worthy. Clean the windows, mirrors, and lights to insure good visibility.

> **Insight** *If you feel comfortable, ask one or more doctors to write a professional letter of recommendation. This will help keep your resume current. Be sure to give them at least two or three weeks so they do not feel pressured.*

Taking Extended Time Off

As mentioned, paid vacation time is not often one of the benefits of traveling. If you work with an agency for a year or so you might ac-crue a week of leave, but that will not be enough time off. Trust me! As a permanent staff member you had to carefully plan your time off especially for Thanksgiving, Christmas, and the New Year. Did you always get them off? You probably had to wait your turn to give everyone an equal chance.

Some facilities expect travelers to fill in for permanent staff during the Holiday period. If this suits your needs, then fine. However traveling gives you the freedom to have any or all the holidays off. If you can afford it you can even take off the entire period from Thanksgiving until after the New Year.

As a traveler you need extended time off to be with family and friends: to rest and recharge yourself. During these times off, unless you work locally, you will not receive a paycheck and your savings will have to sustain you. Your bills will still keep rolling in and you will need money to get to your next travel assignment.

During your months of work, estimate how much you will need to save to ride out those periods of unemployment. Set aside some each payday. This allows you the freedom to take time off when needed, and to negotiate from strength when you are back in the market.

It is possible to time your assignments to end near the Holiday season. If your contract finishes a little too early, you can usually extend for a few weeks to fill in the time closer to when you want to be off. If you wish to work through the Holiday season, specify your required days off within the contract. If the facility finds this unacceptable, and it is really important to you, consider another assignment, or just take the time off.

Given the fact that many travelers want off for the holidays you can imagine the workload chaos this can cause toward the end of the year. But this is just another problem that understaffed facilities have to contend with. And then in January, guess what? Every traveler is ready to return to work! This causes a temporary glut of travelers and you may not get as good an assignment as you wish, or have to wait awhile for an opening. But again, your savings can sustain you through that period and allow you to wait for a good assignment.

Insight — *If you can negotiate some time off, it may be beneficial to start an assignment during the Holiday period. This way you lock in the assignment you want, still get some time off, and avoid the January rush for openings. And if you are willing to work some of the holidays, there will be extra money in it for you. Some facilities offer premium pay during the Holiday season.*

Notes

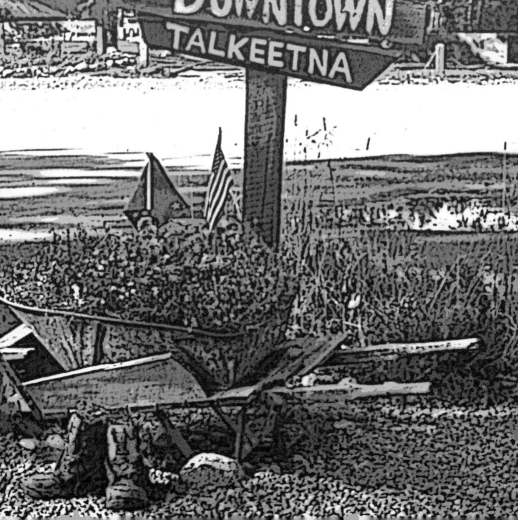

12

Managing Your Money

*Sure, we manage our money.
We "manage" to spend it all!*

Managing your finances on the road need not be difficult. With a little planning and discipline, you should be able to meet your needs, and hopefully all your goals. While everyone's situation is different, there are some basics that apply and can be modified for your individual needs.

Establish Your Financial Game Plan

When we first began traveling I was surprised to find that almost every agency pays their travelers weekly. As a Government employee, I was paid every two weeks. The hospital where my wife worked paid her the same way. While I was delighted to hear of the weekly paycheck, I asked the recruiter about it. Incredibly, she replied that even with the increased income, many travelers live from paycheck to paycheck and need some money coming in weekly to make it. Depending on your situation, over time and with some discipline, you should be able to manage your debt, increase your savings, and not have to live paycheck to paycheck.

Your financial needs as a traveler are about the same as at home but may have to be handled a little differently. You will have to deal with almost everything remotely while on assignment. You can use the phone, e-mail, regular mail, and online banking. We have found we need:

Easy access to cash. In a word, well actually two words, cash back. An ATM card tied to a checking account is hard to beat for instant cash. Many stores allow you to receive cash back with your purchase when using your ATM card. This works well for smaller amounts, say $20 to perhaps $100. Best of all there is no transaction fee. ATM machines are another option. You can hardly walk down a busy street without tripping over at least one. Sure, there are always those little nuisance fees, but even those can be minimized if you shop around, and take larger amounts of money out to reduce the number of transactions.

Easy access to your latest balance and transactions. Any bank worth its salt will provide online banking and a toll-free telephone number as an alternative. This allows you to keep up with your current balances and latest transactions.

Ability to transfer money between accounts. We all have unexpected needs at times that require moving money from one account to another. You need the ability to transfer money between accounts via online banking or a backup toll-free telephone number provided by the bank. While it is sometimes possible to link accounts between banks, we have all of our accounts at one bank. This makes moving money easier via one web site and one login. Be sure to check the fee structure. There should be no charge for transferring money between checking accounts, but there may be a fee associated with transfers from a savings account.

Timely payment of bills. Unfortunately your bills continue even when you travel. Many people take advantage of the bill paying service at their bank. We prefer to use direct debit for those bills that are the same, or nearly the same, each month. We write checks for the other bills that are not well suited for direct debit.

Based on the above, your bank should have these characteristics:

* A full service FDIC bank that provides checking accounts (with an ATM debit card) and savings accounts.

* Online banking capabilities to allow you to view the balances, recent transactions, and transfer between accounts. It should also have a toll free telephone number as a backup if you suddenly lose web access.

* Bill paying capability.

Fortunately, most banks today provide these necessary services free or at a minimal charge. You probably have at least the basics set up already.

> **Insight**
>
> *We use a regional bank with all the above services. On those rare occasions when we receive a personal check, and are unable to cash it locally, we just write "For Deposit Only" on the back, put the account number on it, and mail it to our home town bank for deposit into our account.*

With direct deposit, an ATM card, and online banking, we have no need for a local bank account while on assignment. By the way, as of this writing there is no bank that has branches in all 50 states.

If your bank does not provide the capabilities above, shop around for one that does. Granted you will have to buy new checks, get a new debit card, change your direct deposit, etc., but it will be worth it in the long run. When you're on the road, your finances need to be as simple and accessible as possible.

Setting Up Your Accounts

Be aware of security issues when setting up your accounts. You can't be too careful in this age of identity theft and database intrusions. It is certainly possible to set up one account dealing with all your checks, ATM, direct debit, and even emergency savings, but if this account is illegally accessed, you could find yourself in financial hardship until the situation is resolved. We prefer to separate our money into different accounts to increase security purposes, and for better accountability, but all under the same bank for convenience.

We have found that establishing three accounts at our home town regional FDIC bank satisfies our needs:

* **First account.** A full service primary checking account with an ATM card tied to it. Paychecks are deposited directly into this account. This is used for daily living requirements.

* **Second account.** A checking account used for direct debits to pay most bills. We do not buy checks for this account. We have an ATM card attached to it but only for emergency purposes if a problem develops in accessing our first account. Direct debits are used to pay bills that are fixed (or nearly fixed) each month. Your home mortgage, car payment, utilities and insurance items are just a few candidates. Just be sure this account has enough money each month to cover the debits. Bills not possible or too inconvenient to pay by direct debit, are paid by check from the first account. **Caution:** Do not plan to use a savings account for direct debits. While most companies have no problem, some cannot deduct from a savings account. Also, your bank may impose a fee for transactions and may limit

the number of transactions from a savings account. If you are not supporting a permanent home and do not have a lot of monthly bills, this special debit checking account may not be necessary. You may want to pay your few bills directly from your primary checking account.

❊ **Third account.** A savings account for cash savings and emergency funds. This is where all excess money goes each payday. You may have to move some money back into your other accounts from time to time but put as much money as you can into savings each payday and leave it alone for as long as possible. This will have to sustain you during your time off.

> **Insight** *If you are saving for a particular purpose, say to buy a new car, consider opening a separate savings account for it. That way you are less likely to withdraw the money for routine expenses.*

By separating your money into several accounts you can increase your security and keep better track of where it goes.

And while you are setting money aside, don't forget to contribute to your 401(k). After all, you don't want to work forever, do you? (Wow, what a great lead-in to the next chapter!)

Notes

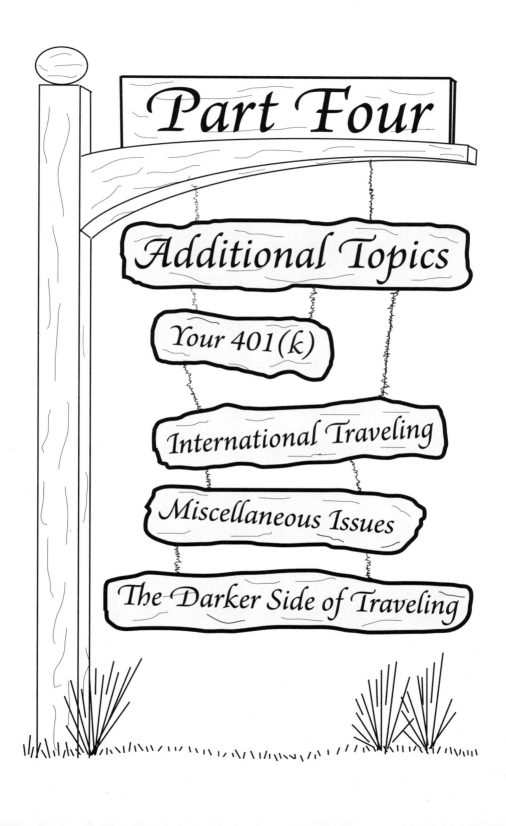

Part Four

Additional Topics

Your 401(k)

International Traveling

Miscellaneous Issues

The Darker Side of Traveling

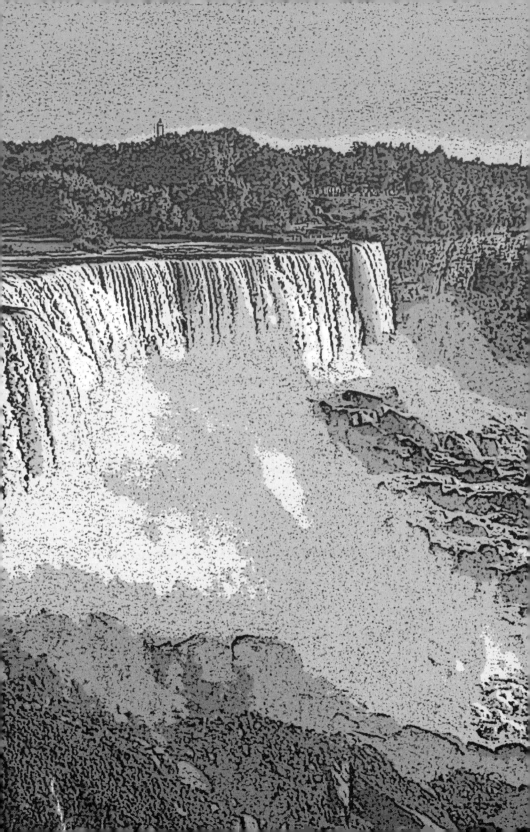

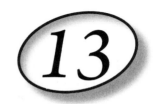

Your 401(k)

*Gather five financial advisors together and what do
you get? At least six opinions.*

*R*etirement

That word has a nice ring, doesn't it? No more 10 or 12 hour shifts.
No more working weekends! Time to spend doing what **you** want:
relax, your hobbies, visit your family . . . whatever.

So how will you finance your life after work? Do you plan to win the
lottery? Is your Uncle Bill going to leave you a bundle? Will your kids
support you? Oh, I know, you're going to depend on Social Security!
Well, you know where this is going. If you have not already, you need
to take responsibility to plan and invest for your retirement.

If you are actively participating in your agency's retirement plan,
congratulations! You are doing yourself the biggest favor possible.
If you have not joined, now is the time! Why now? You can't afford
to wait any longer. The sooner you start, the more time your money
will have to grow. Even a small amount invested regularly can make

a big difference. Planning for life after work can mean the difference between an enjoyable retirement lifestyle and one that just gets by.

Excuses . . . Excuses

If you have delayed joining your 401(k) program, do any of these sound familiar?

- ✳ *I can't afford to save.*
- ✳ *I don't understand investing.*
- ✳ *I'm worried about losing my money.*
- ✳ *The forms are too complicated.*
- ✳ *I'm too old to start.*
- ✳ *My money is not accessible until I retire.*
- ✳ *I change agencies too often.*

I can't afford to save. I know money is tight. It's always tight. But you find ways to juggle and pay your bills. If you are like the rest of us, sometimes you have to scrimp on some items to keep your bills under control. Here's an idea: pay yourself just as you would pay a bill. And pay yourself first by having the amount deducted automatically from your pay before you have a chance to spend it!

Start out slowly with a small amount: perhaps $50 per week, and increase it slowly over time. Still think you can't afford it? Come on, be honest. Can you eat less often at your favorite restaurant? Do you really need that expensive watch or purse? If you are honest you can think of a number of ways to reduce your expenditures just enough to help insure your financial future.

You may think that $50 a week is not enough to make a difference. But when you think of it as $2600 per year it becomes a little more meaningful. Even investing a small amount can have a significant result over time. Historically the stock market has returned about 10% per year. And this isn't just the good years either! This includes the crash of 1929, the Great Depression, and many downturns since, some lasting several years.

But let's not even assume a return of 10% on your money. Let's use 8%. If you invest $50 per week for 30 years at 8% you should have approximately $312,000. (If you use the historical 10% return you should have about $468,000 after that same 30 years.) And saving more per week can have an even larger payback over time.

I don't understand investing. For a new investor the choices offered by your 401(k) plan can be dizzying. Even the terminology can be intimidating. Your plan should offer a broad range of investment options with different risk and return characteristics: from more conservative choices to those that are more aggressive. The material should also help identify what type of investor you are, and which choices may be appropriate for you. If you're uncomfortable choosing your investment options, you may want to opt for several that are more conservative and have a lower level of risk. Your agency or 401(k) administrator may offer financial counseling to help you get started. As you become more knowledgeable, you can rearrange your investments to better suite your investing style.

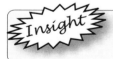 *It's more important to get started than to pick the absolute correct allocation initially. In fact there is no "perfect" allocation.*

I'm worried about losing my money. This is where being a long term investor helps. You need to have the discipline to ride out short term market downturns to give your account a chance to grow. Granted, you may have to re-evaluate your allocation during those periods, but not participating or keeping your money in ultra conservative choices will not allow you to meet your long term financial needs.

The forms are too complicated. Come on! As a healthcare worker you fill out forms all day. Contact your plan administrator if you need clarification.

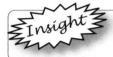 Some plans allow you to sign-up and choose your options completely online thus eliminating the need to fill out any forms.

I'm too old to start. Not necessarily. Even if you are just a few years from retirement there are tax advantages to saving through a Traditional 401(k). Each year your taxable income can be reduced by your contributions. You might be surprised by the gains that only a few years of growth can produce. And when you withdraw the money you may be in a lower tax bracket.

My money is not accessible until I retire. True, your 401(k) is designed as a long term retirement program. However, some plans allow you to borrow from your account. Please avoid this unless absolutely necessary. Leave your money in your account and give it a chance to grow. Withdrawals in the case of hardship may also be available. As with loans, withdrawals should be avoided. Taxes and the early withdrawal penalty can take close to 1/3 of your withdrawal.

I change agencies too often. It is a hassle to enroll with every new agency but your retirement is too important not to follow through. You can consolidate your old 401(k) plans by rolling them over to an Individual Retirement Account (IRA). This reduces your number of accounts and often allows more investment options.

No more excuses. The time for action is now. If you don't have a recent 401(k) information packet from your agency, call and request one. It will have everything you need to get started.

401(k) Overview

Many workers have their retirement under "defined benefit plans". These plans are usually offered by larger companies and are often the result of labor union bargaining over many years. The company sets money aside as part of the worker's pay package. When the worker retires they receive a pension based on a wage formula and years worked. Often medical benefits are part of the retirement package.

Defined benefit plans are a dying breed. Companies with these plans have felt the effect on their bottom line as retirees live longer and medical costs continue to rise. Today they seem to be using every device to reduce, or even eliminate this growing long term burden.

From the worker's standpoint there are at least two problems with defined benefit plans. Some workers change jobs too often to accumulate enough time to retire from any one company, and some smaller companies cannot afford the cost associated with such a plan. This left many workers without a true retirement plan and having to depend on their savings and Social Security in their retirement years.

In 1981, Congress established the 401(k) program to encourage long term retirement savings. Under the program your employer can deduct a specified amount of money each payday, and deposit it into your 401(k) account. Your money is placed in investment options you choose from those offered through the plan. Some employers will match your contribution up to a certain percentage. This match is sometimes held in a separate account and becomes yours once you are vested. Vesting refers to the waiting period before the agency's match amount becomes legally yours. Some agencies allow you to be vested immediately. Others may require employment for a specific period of time prior to taking ownership of the match amount. Your 401(k) is also "portable". When you change jobs you can take it with you. Because it is a long term retirement program early withdrawals are discouraged. In general you cannot withdraw money until you are 59-1/2 without incurring a 10% penalty.

Many companies have converted to the 401(k) program, shifting the responsibility of retirement to their employees. Even the Federal Government revised its retirement plan in the mid-1980's to be more in line with the 401(k) scenario.

Two versions of the 401(k) program currently exist: Traditional and Roth. Your agency may not offer both.

Traditional 401(k). This is the original version which most agencies offer. It allows "before tax" contributions. The amount you set aside each pay period is deducted from your taxable wages thus reducing your tax burden for that year. If you earn $60,000 in taxable wages and contribute $5,000 to your 401(k) during the year, you will owe taxes on $55,000. Instant tax relief!

Your account grows tax deferred. No taxes are due until the money is withdrawn, hopefully many years later. By then you may be in a lower tax bracket. Since your contributions were not taxed originally, the full amount of any withdrawal is taxable: contributions and proceeds. You must begin withdrawing your money by age 70-1/2.

Roth 401(k). This more recent version allows "after tax" contributions to be made to your account. There is no immediate tax benefit, but the proceeds grow tax-free. This is especially appealing to younger investors with a long time horizon. Since your contributions have already been taxed, the full amount of any withdrawal is tax free: contributions and proceeds. There is no requirement to withdraw your money from a Roth 401(k) plan. In fact, you can leave the account to your heirs.

Both the Traditional and the Roth are designed as long term retirement programs. Again, with only a few exceptions you can not withdraw your money until age 59-1/2 without incurring a 10% penalty.

Contribution limits. There is a limit to the amount you can contribute each year to your 401(k). In 2007 it was $15,500. In 2008 the limit began to be indexed for inflation in $500 increments. Employees who are at least fifty years old can contribute an additional "catch up" amount. In 2007 this amount was $5000. In 2008, this also began to be indexed for inflation in $500 increments. Your 401(k) plan administrator can tell you the limits for each year.

Your agency may not offer both Traditional and Roth 401(k), but if they do, you can choose the best fit given your age and outlook on taxes. If your program permits, you can even allocate your contribution between both plans. You can defer some taxes now while allowing the other portion to grow tax-free. Keep in mind your combined contributions cannot exceed the yearly maximum.

Congressional action now permits employers to enroll their employees automatically. The employee must "opt out" to decline participation. It is hoped this will encourage enrollment and allow more workers to benefit from this important long term retirement plan.

Insight *If you are negotiating with a new agency and find they do not offer a 401(k), or there is a prolonged waiting period to join, consider dropping them and negotiating with an agency that better meets your needs. If you have an existing contract with an agency that does not offer a 401(k), consider changing agencies as soon as your contract ends . . . and tell them why you are changing. Yes, your retirement is that important!!*

Common 401(k) Mistakes

Not enrolling. As mentioned, many continually delay joining their 410(k). Excuses abound but the fact is you have to look out for your own future. No one else will. The sooner you start, the more time your money will have to grow.

Taking too little risk. Some are too conservative in their investment choices. If you have a long time horizon you can ride out the market downturns and should have a good return over time. It's alright to invest a smaller portion of your account in a more conservative choice. This can add stability especially during volatile periods in the stock market. However, many experts stress the longer your time horizon, the more you should have in stock mutual funds to achieve the growth necessary to meet your goals.

Taking too much risk. At the opposite end of the scale are those that shoot for superior gains every year by being in the most aggressive choices in their 401(k). Market downturns can quickly sweep away gains from previous years. And it can take years for your account to recover. You can moderate your exposure to sudden drops by diversifying through several investment choices and still have a chance for good returns over the long term.

Missing out on the agency match. If your agency provides matching funds, try to contribute enough to qualify for the maximum match amount. After all, this is free money.

Borrowing against your account. Some plans allow you to take out loans against your account. Emergencies happen, but you should borrow only as an absolute last resort. Not only do you lose the growth on that money during the loan period, but the repayment is made with "after tax" dollars. Then, if you have a traditional 401(k), when you ultimately remove the money at retirement that same money is taxed again!

Cashing out. Travelers tend to change agencies fairly often. When you leave, one of the worst things you can do is cash out your account. Between taxes and penalties you will probably end up with about 2/3 of your money. Better to leave it with the agency (if you like the investment choices and your agency allows it), or roll it over to an IRA.

Plan of Action

Enroll. Your agency may or may not enroll you automatically. Call your plan administrator and request a recent 401(k) packet. It will have the necessary forms and available investment options. It may also provide assistance in determining which investments are appropriate given the number of years until retirement and your tolerance to risk.

Decide how much to set aside each payday. Many have difficulty deciding how much they can afford to save. Start slowly and increase the amount over time as you become more comfortable with this reduced take home pay. You will probably find yourself wanting to save more once you see your account building and realize how painless the process is.

Choose your investment options and allocation. If you are new to investing, choosing investment options and deciding how much to allocate to each is the most difficult task. And, sadly, it deters many from joining. The plan material should contain guidance on how to evaluate your investing temperament and make the appropriate choices. Many experts recommend maintaining a diversified portfolio consisting of stock and bond mutual funds.

For the Novice :
Choosing Your Initial Investments

Read through the materials provided by your agency and learn as much as you can, but don't get bogged down in details that seem obscure. There is plenty of time later to understand more. Just try to get a broad overview at this time.

If you really do not have a clue as to what your initial allocation should be, many financial advisors suggest one of a series of funds called "Lifecycle", "Lifestyle", "Target" (or a similar name) that has a retirement year associated with each. They usually run in five year increments from five years to forty years away. For instance, a Life-cycle 2035 fund is aimed for those retiring near the year 2035. They are billed as one stop investment shopping. Each lifecycle fund is made up of a diversified mixture of large and small company stocks, bonds, international stocks, fixed income investments, etc. The fund managers adjust the allocation as time progresses: becoming more conservative as the retirement date approaches. Lifecycle 2020 is more conservative than Lifecycle 2045.

If you feel most comfortable with this option, choose the lifecycle fund with the date closest to your expected retirement date as your investment choice. Keep in mind this is just to get you started. As you become more knowledgeable about investing you can remain invested in the fund or choose your own mix of investments.

Next enter the amount you wish to contribute each pay period and that you want 100% of your contributions to go to that fund. If you are not sure how much you can afford to save, start off slowly (say $50) and increase your contribution over time.

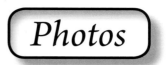

Photos

During our years of traveling we have taken thousands of photographs: from Boston to Seattle, from Georgia to Alaska. And a lot of stops in between!

Here are a few of our favorites. Believe me it was hard to choose a few from the many. Each one represents memories of our stay or of our traveling to and from assignments.

One of the great benefits of being a traveler is to visit many of the historic and scenic places of America you have only heard about, and often to stay long enough to really enjoy the area.

If you are a traveler, or decide to travel, be sure to pack your camera for each assignment.

We hope you enjoy this photo section. For us there is really no other place on earth like America. And maybe these will help entice you to join us "on the road"!

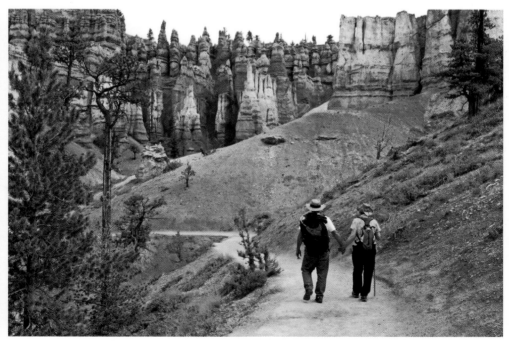

Barry and Donna Padgett hiking among the Hoodoos in Bryce Canyon, Utah

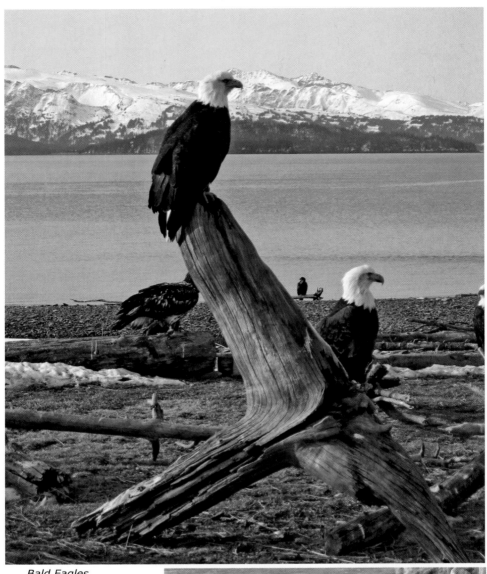
Bald Eagles,
Homer Spit, Alaska

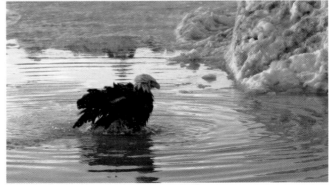
Bald Eagle taking a
VERY COLD bath at
Homer Spit

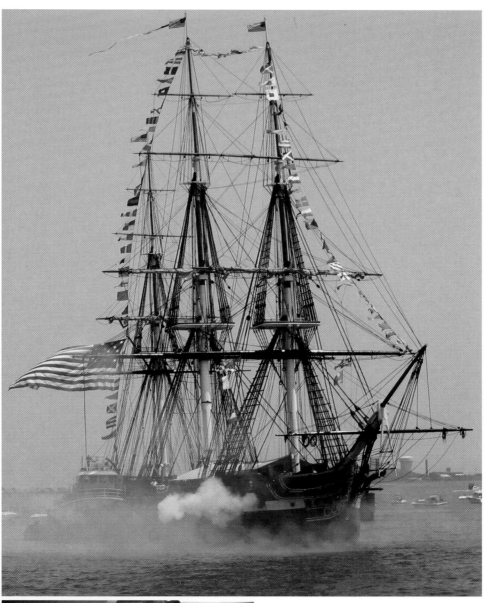

The USS Constitution ("Old Ironsides") fires a 21 gun salute in Boston Harbor during a 4th of July celebration.

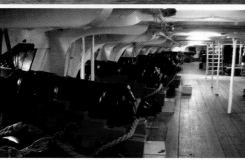

The canon deck of "Old Ironsides".

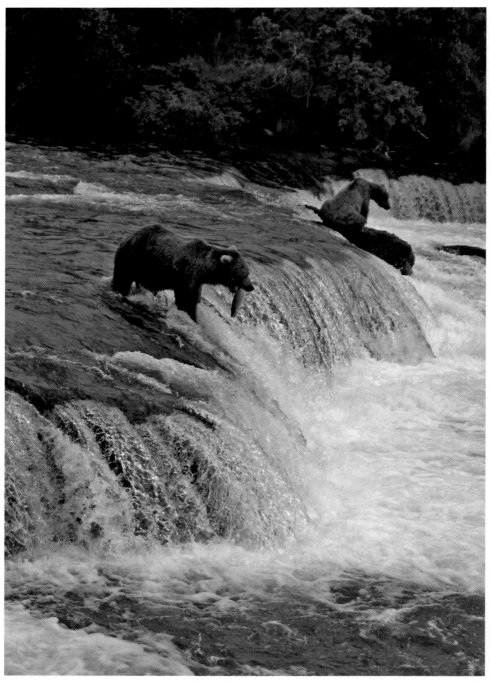

Brown Bears feasting on silver salmon, Brooks Falls, Katmai National Preserve, Alaska

Each summer the salmon swim upstream to their spawning grounds. They must jump the falls to continue their journey . . . and the bears are waiting.

Evening Glow - Sierra Vista, Arizona

San Francisco - The Sea Lions of Fisherman's Wharf began appearing several years ago. Because they were destroying the docks, the local authorities tried several measures to discourage them from staying. Eventually the sea lions prevailed and were allocated their own area. And as you can see they are quite a tourist attraction.

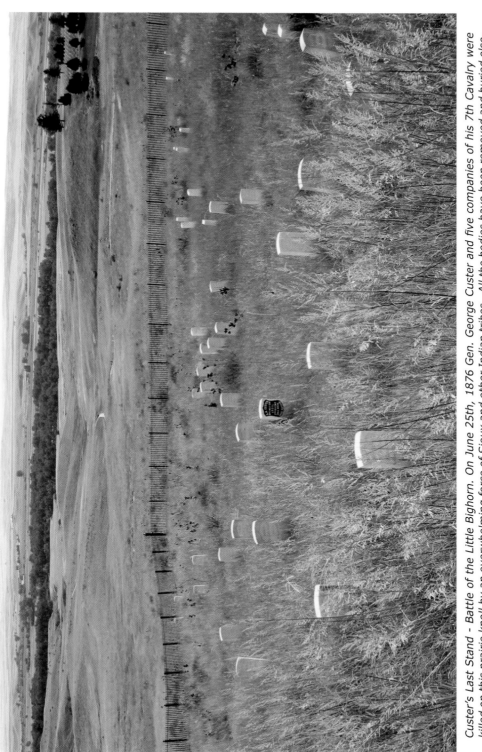

Custer's Last Stand - Battle of the Little Bighorn. On June 25th, 1876 Gen. George Custer and five companies of his 7th Cavalry were killed on this prairie knoll by an overwhelming force of Sioux and other Indian tribes . All the bodies have been removed and buried else-where. The markers indicate where each fell. The marker with the black shield is where Gen. Custer died.

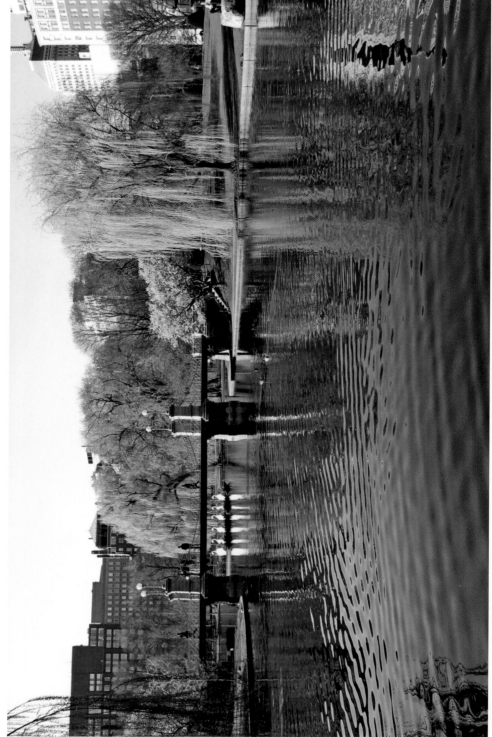

Early Spring at Boston's Public Garden

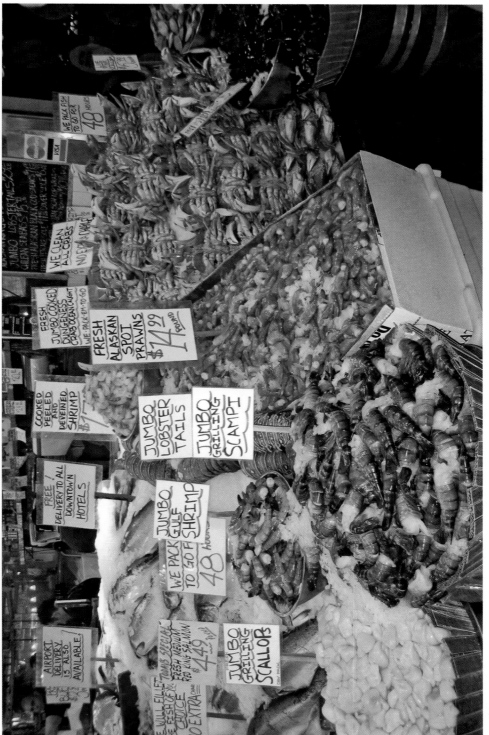

Fresh seafood, meats, fruits, and vegetables abound at Pike Street Market in Seattle.

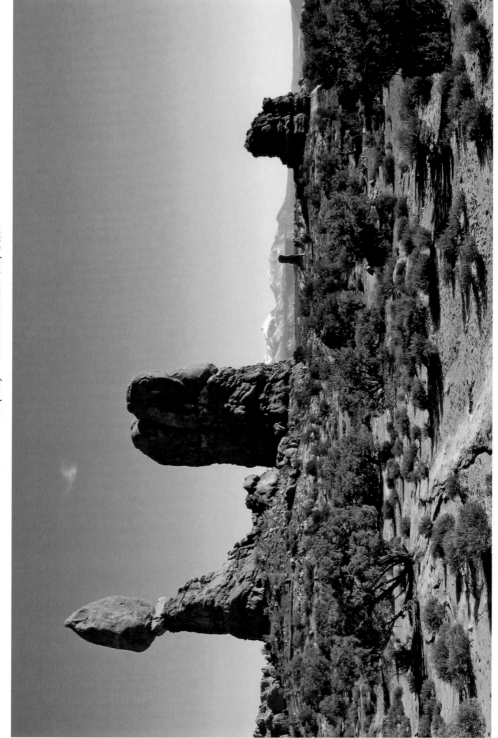

Balanced Rock (left) - Arches National Park, Utah

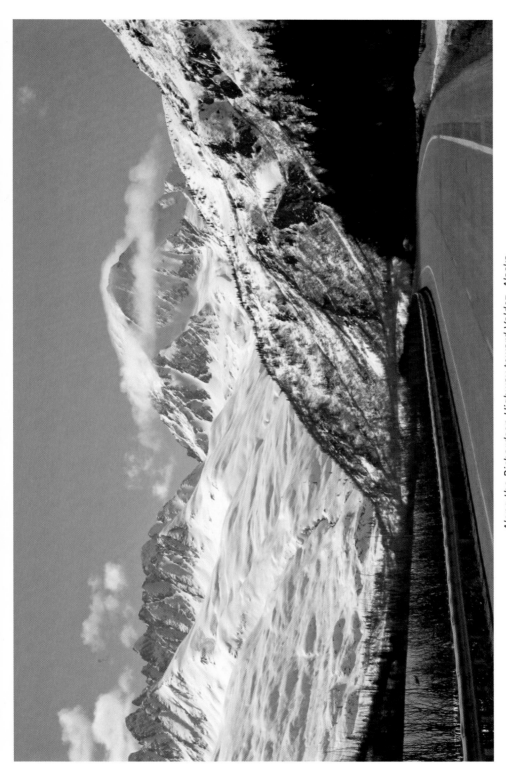

Along the Richardson Highway toward Valdez, Alaska

Morning sky over Colby, Kansas

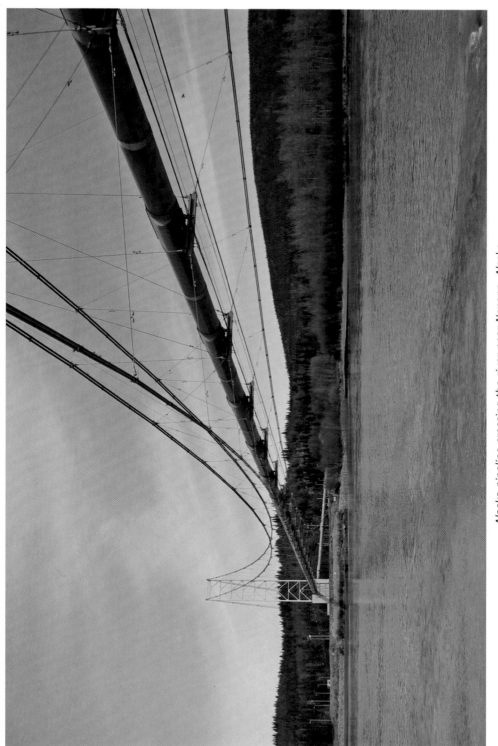

Alaska pipeline crossing the river near Nenana, Alaska

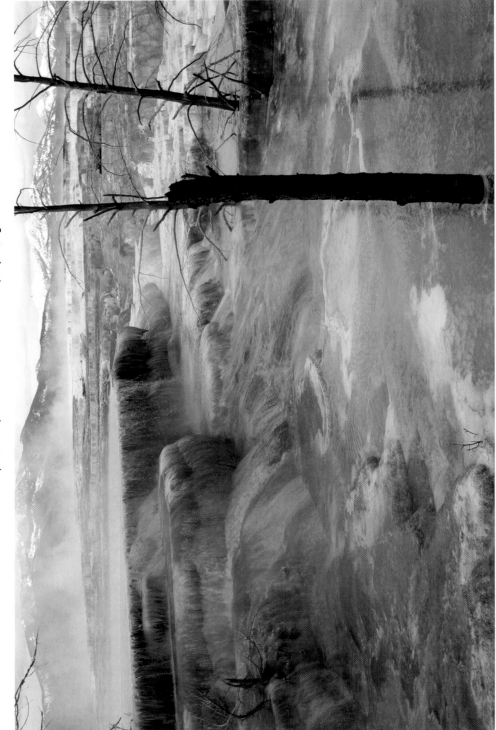

Sulphur flow, Yellowstone National Park, Wyoming

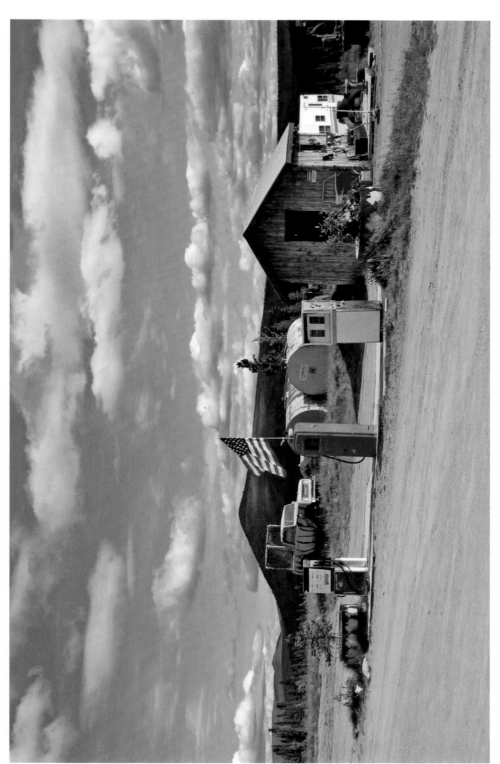

Gas station near the Alaska - Canada border - Top of the World Highway

Landscape at the Top of the World Highway. You can see how it got its name!

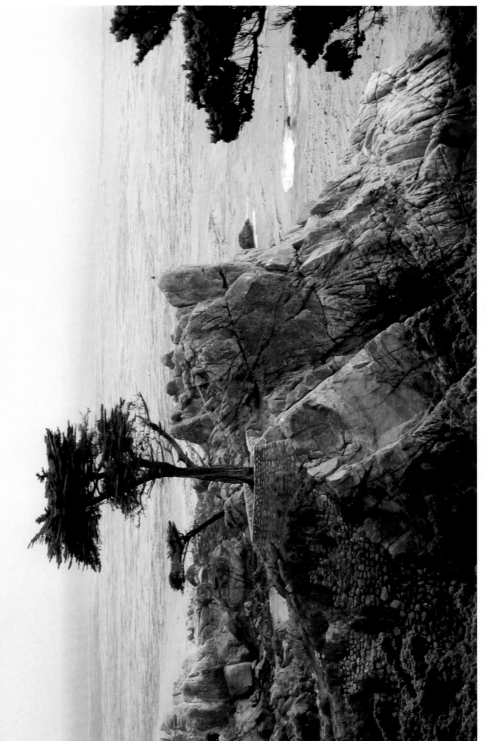

Lone Pine Tree - Monterey Bay, California

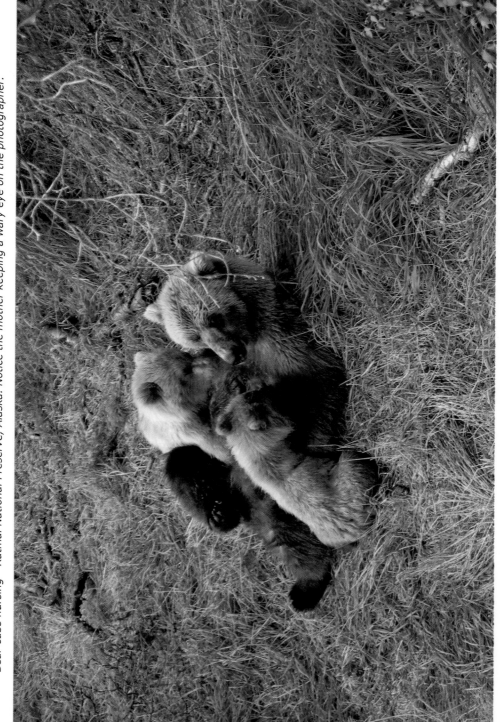

Bear cubs nursing - Katmai National Preserve, Alaska. Notice the mother keeping a wary eye on the photographer.

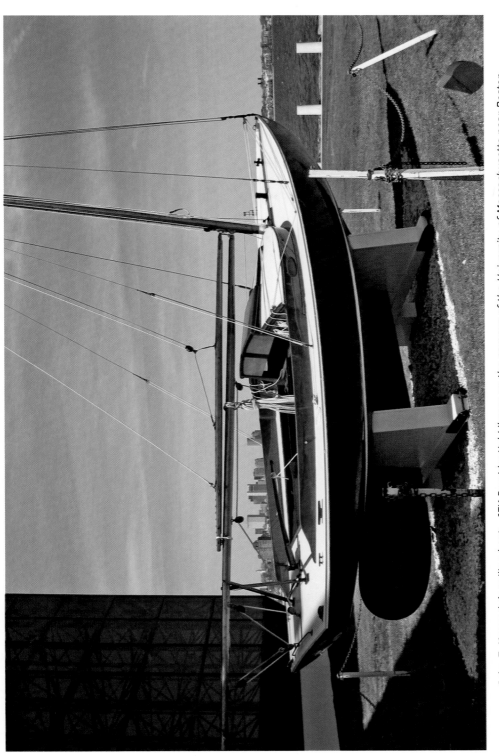

John F. Kennedy's sailing boat - JFK Presidential Library on the campus of the University of Massachusetts near Boston

British soldiers rush to formation at the re-enactment of the Battle of Lexington, Lexington, Massachusetts.

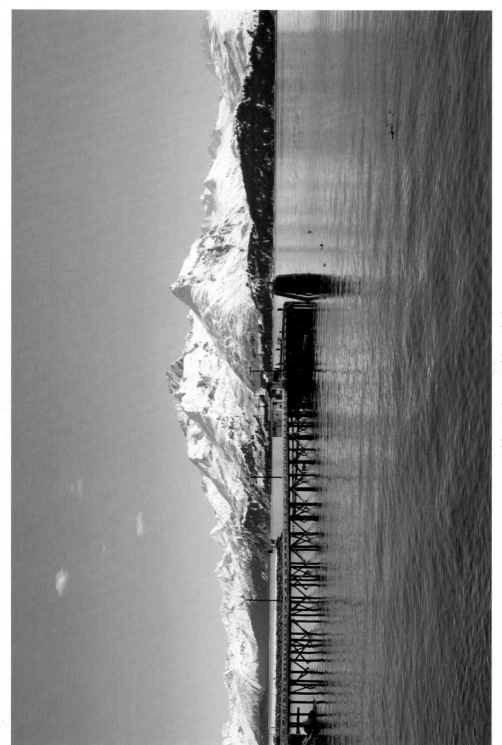

Valdez Harbor - Valdez, Alaska

Hoodoos at the "Silent City" - Bryce Canyon National Park, Utah

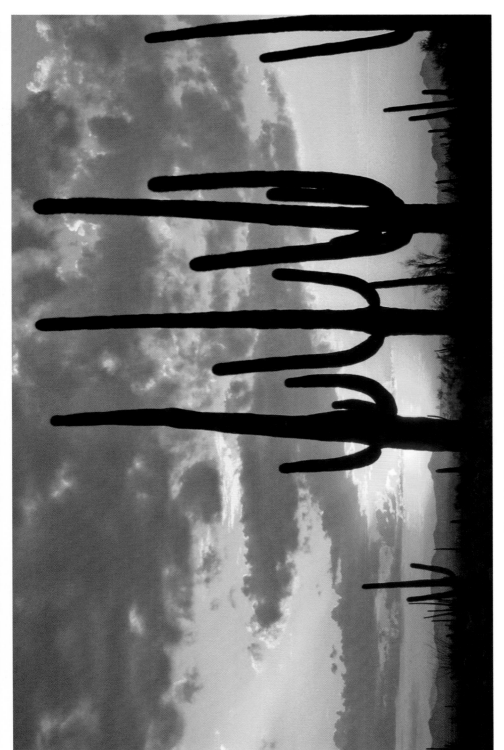

Sunset in Saguaro National Park near Tucson, Arizona

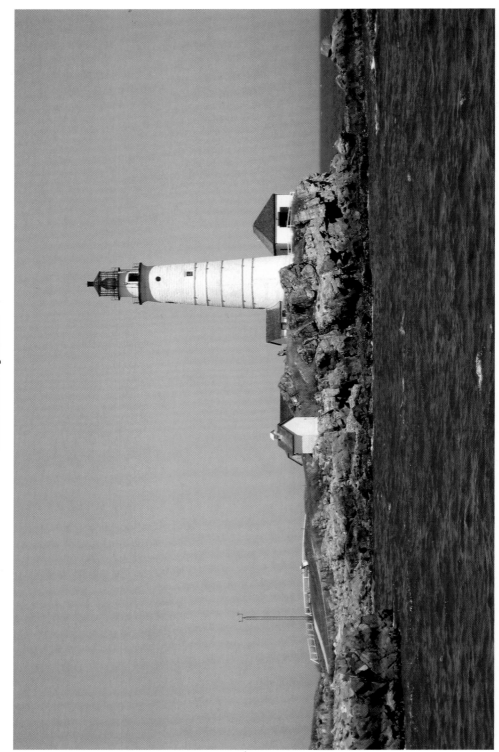

Boston Harbor Lighthouse

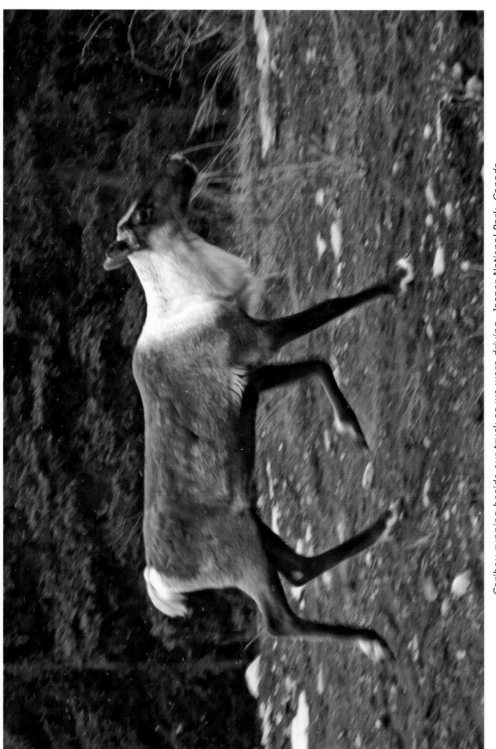

Caribou running beside our truck as we were driving- Jasper National Park, Canada

Stone logs - Petrified Forest National Park, Arizona

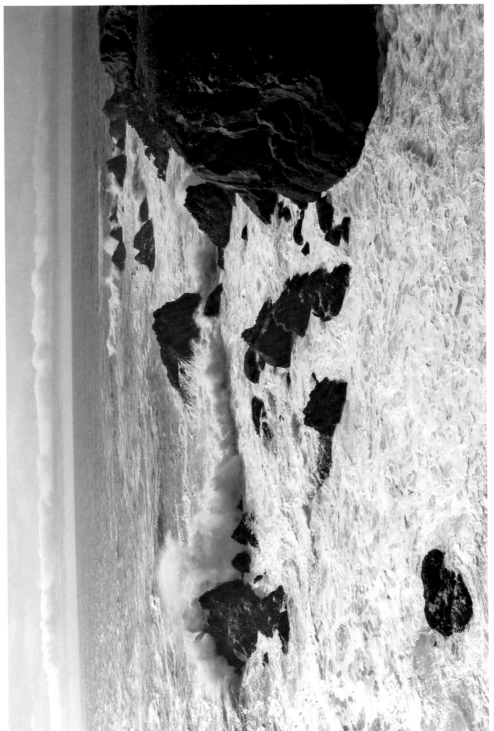

Stillwater Cove, Coast of Northern California

Ruth Glacier, Mt. McKinley (Denali), Alaska

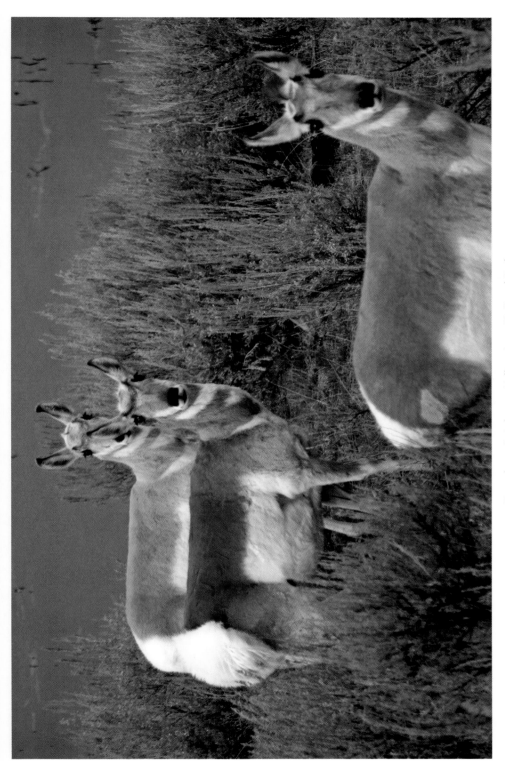

Pronghorn Antelope - Yellowstone National Park

Autumn across the Palmer Hay Flats toward Pioneer Peak - Palmer, Alaska

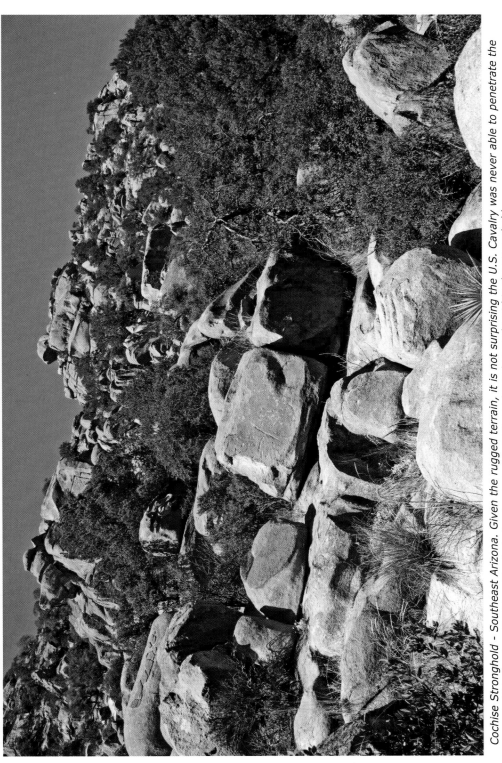

Cochise Stronghold - Southeast Arizona. Given the rugged terrain, it is not surprising the U.S. Cavalry was never able to penetrate the stronghold to capture Cochise. He died of natural causes and was buried secretly within the stronghold.

Polar Bear pushing a ball - Alaska Zoo, Anchorage, Alaska

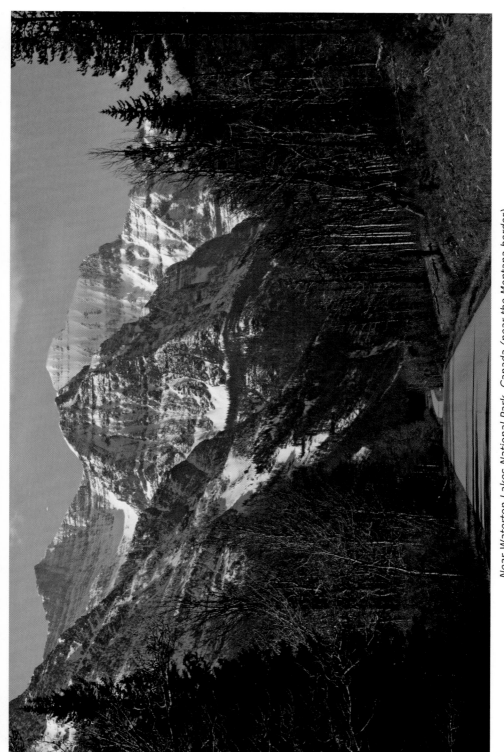

Near Waterton Lakes National Park, Canada (near the Montana border)

Painted Desert, Northern Arizona

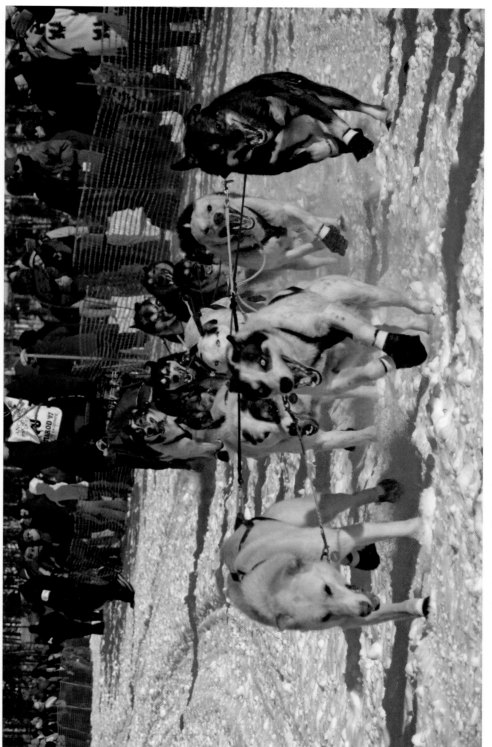

The dogs are exited and eager to get going - Start of the Iditarod Race, Willow Lake, Alaska

Buggy Whip cactus in bloom - Sedona, Arizona

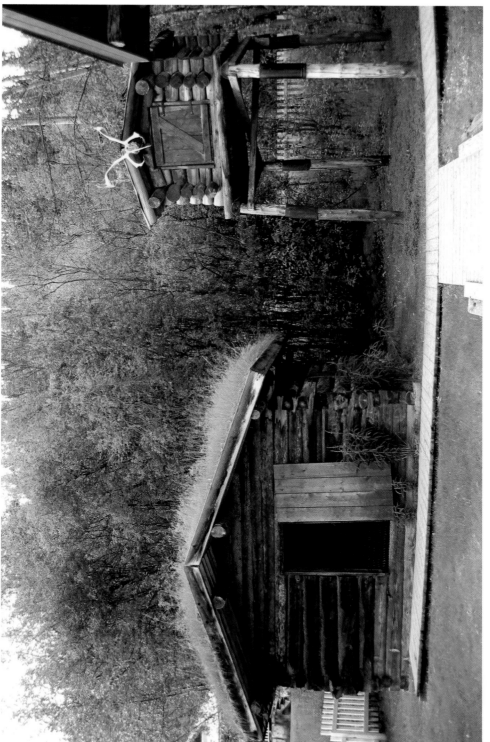

Jack London's cabin (author of "Call of the Wild") - Dawson, Yukon Territory

Denali (Mt. McKinley) on a rare clear day. Near Talkeetna, Alaska

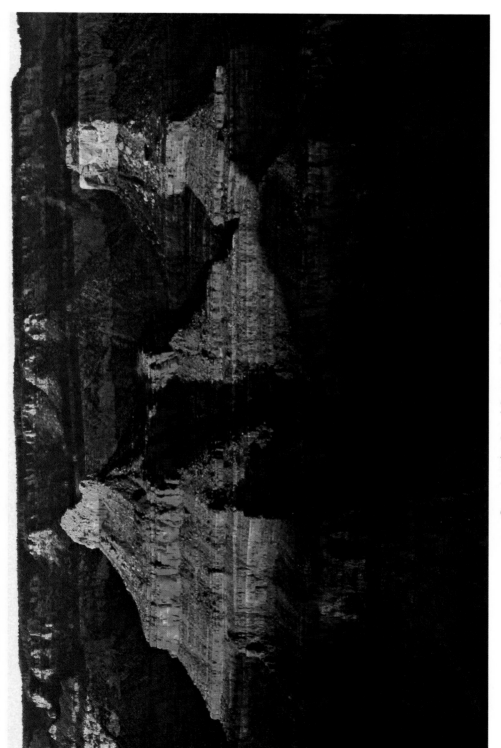

Sunset at the Grand Canyon National Park, Arizona

Anchorage, Alaska at dusk.

Breaking the bank - Las Vegas, Nevada

American Falls, Niagara Falls, New York

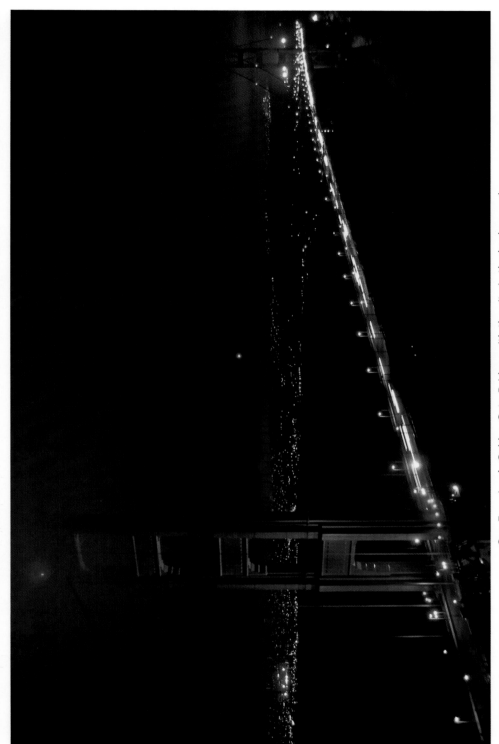

San Francisco's Golden Gate Bridge, with the city in the background

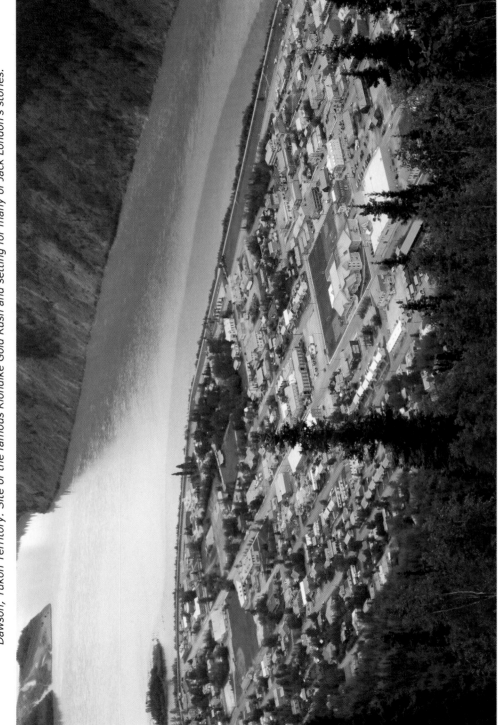

Dawson, Yukon Territory. Site of the famous Klondike Gold Rush and setting for many of Jack London's stories.

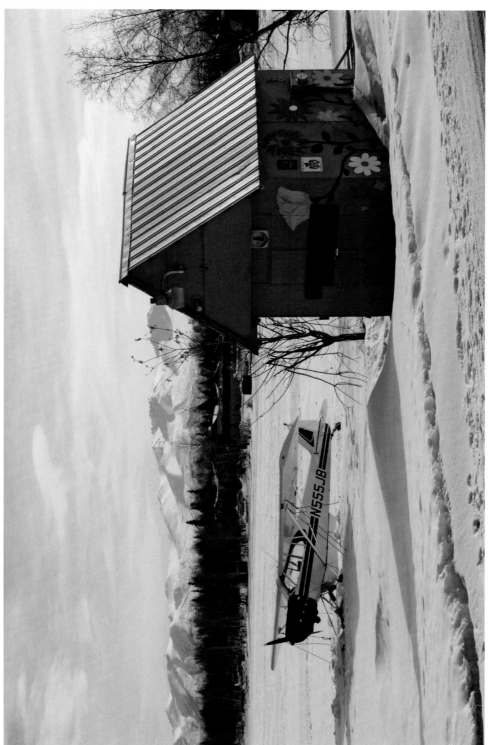

Float plane and storage house at Lake Hood - Anchorage, Alaska

Boulder Dam and Lake Mead near Las Vegas

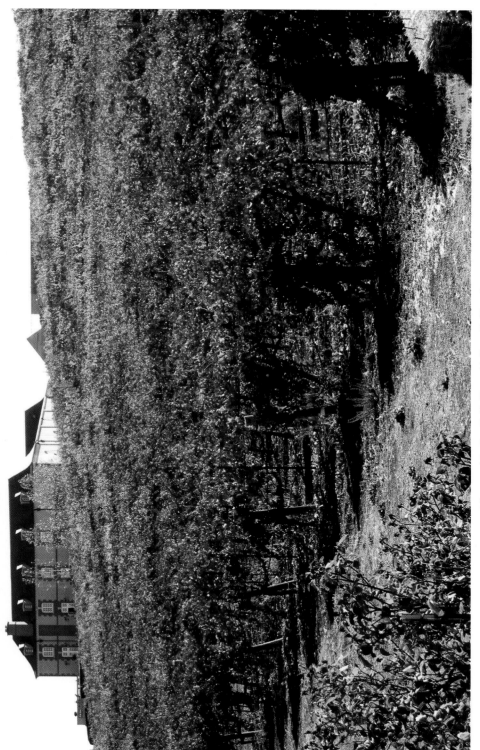

Vineyard in the Fall. Napa Valley, California

Young Elk - Yellowstone National Park, Wyoming

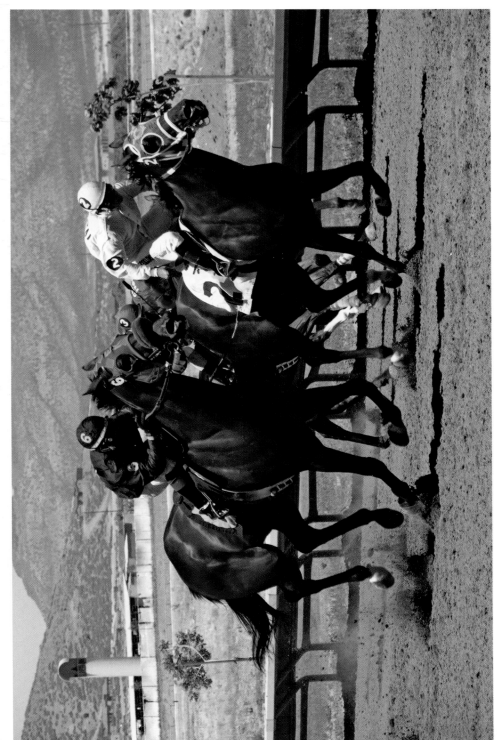

Horse racing - Yavapai Downs, Prescott, Arizona

Buffalo at the Grand Teton National Park, Wyoming

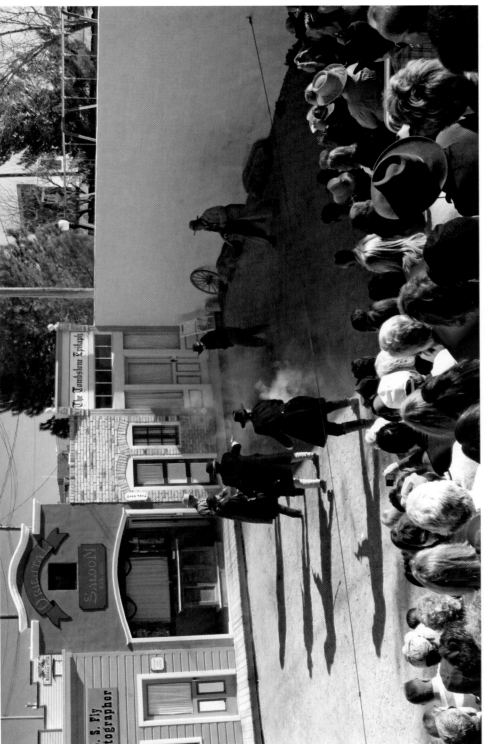

Re-enactment of the famous "Gunfight at the OK Corral", Tombstone, Arizona

Airport at Palmer, Alaska

Chinatown, San Francisco

Autumn back road, central Vermont

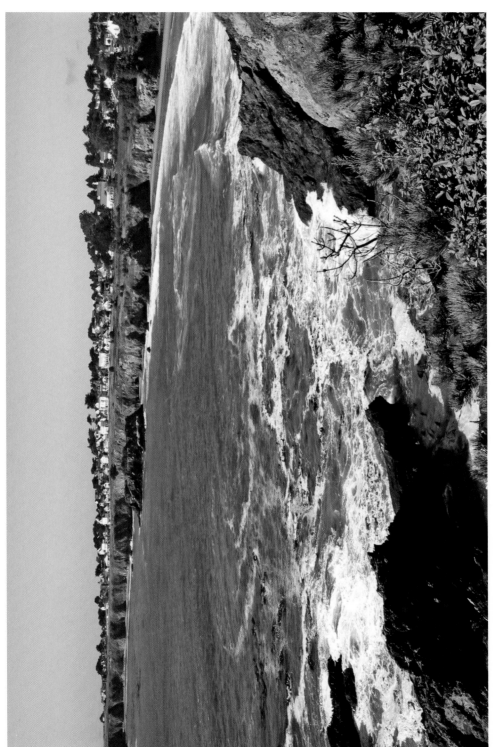

Mendocino, Northern California

New York City's East River and Manhattan Island during the Sunset Cruise

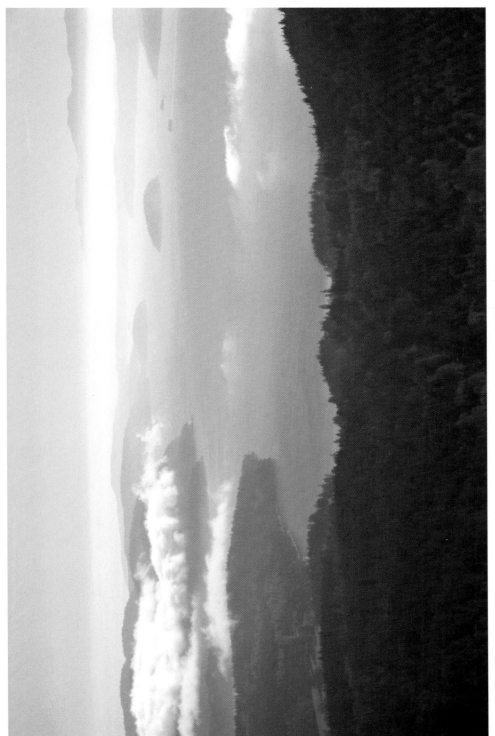

Misty Morning in the San Juan Islands near Seattle

Luther Burbank's Home and Gardens, Santa Rosa, California

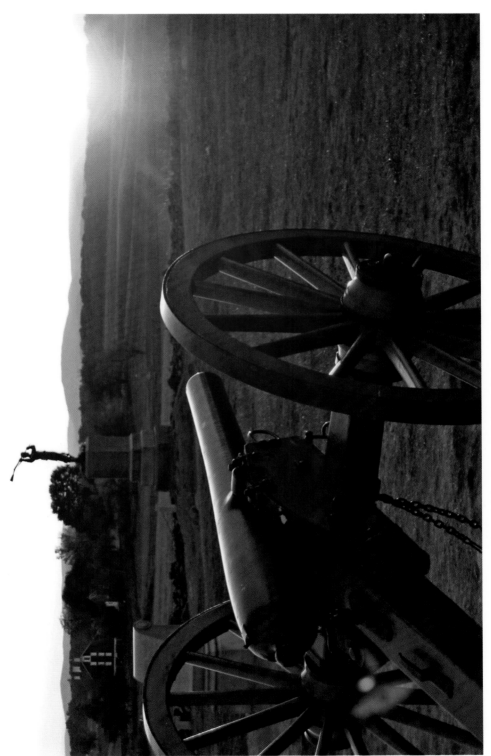

Scene of the famous Pickett's Charge, Gettysburg, Pennsylvania

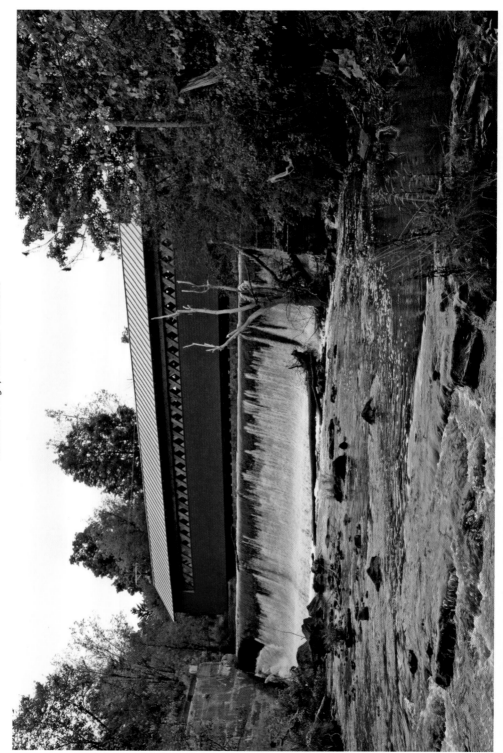

Covered bridge, southern Vermont

Smoky Mountains, North Georgia

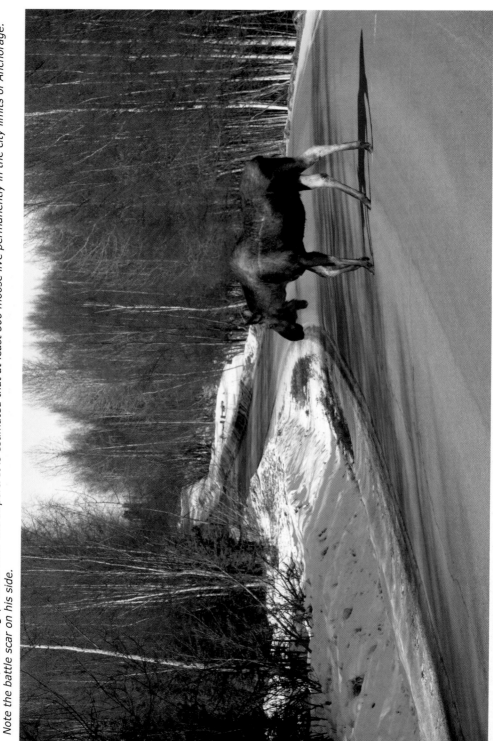

Male moose, Anchorage, Alaska near the airport. It is estimated that at least 300 moose live permanently in the city limits of Anchorage. Note the battle scar on his side.

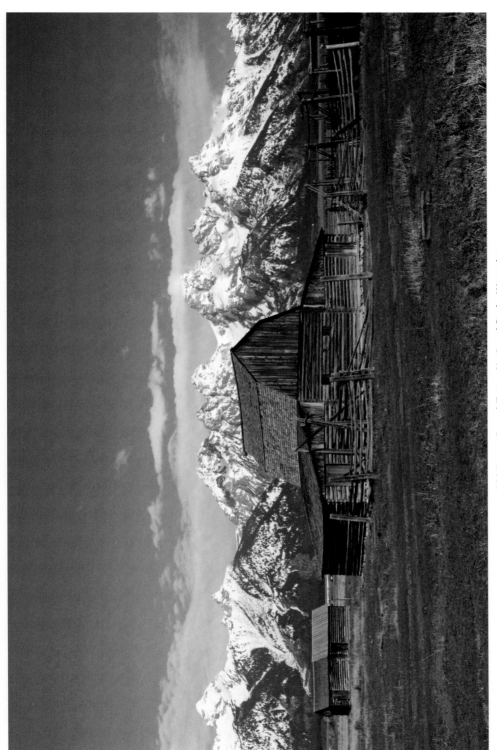

Old Barn, Grand Teton National Park, Wyoming

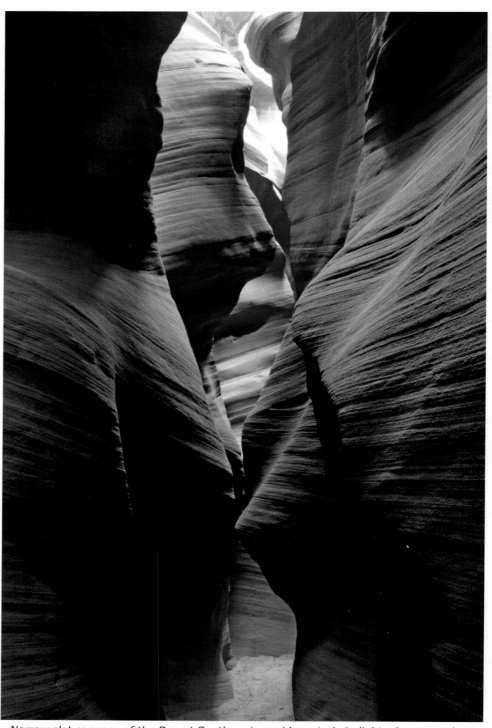

Narrow slot canyons of the Desert Southwest provide a study in light, shapes, and texture. This one is near Page, Arizona.

Insight
Lifecycle funds can be a good choice for the novice, or those that want to put their investments on automatic pilot. Even if you choose this option take the time to become more knowledgeable about the market and your investment temperament. You may be better served long term by choosing your own mix of investments.

Determining Your Investment Temperament

What kind of investor are you? Are you willing to take some risk for a greater potential gain or are you more conservative, wishing to minimize the effect of market downturns. Your time horizon and risk tolerance can be used to determine your investment profile or "temperament".

Your time horizon. This refers to the amount of time remaining until you retire and begin withdrawing your account. Most use age 62 or 65 for planning purposes. If you are 30 and plan to retire at 65 you have a time horizon of 35 years. However, you must also take into account your expected longevity. If you have a family history of living longer you will need to plan your investments accordingly. Even if you begin withdrawing your money at age 62 or 65 you may need at least some money in higher growth areas to provide extra income during your retirement years. The last thing you want is to run out of money in your final remaining years.

Your risk tolerance. This concept is very important but difficult for new investors to determine. It refers to how well you can psychologically tolerate short-term market downturns. It requires honesty and soul-searching on your part. While others can give advice and guidance, only you can ultimately decide your level of tolerance.

Again, the overall historical return of the modern stock market in good times and bad is about 10% per year. Sounds good doesn't it? Long term investors have been able to ride out the short term downturns and have a good return over the long term. The question is, do you have the stomach to hang in there when the stock market goes down for extended periods? At first blush you might think, "Sure. I know the market will eventually recover." But let's consider an example.

Suppose your account has been invested mostly in stocks for about 10 years and you have a total of $50,000. Your returns have varied but overall have been good. Things are rolling along well. Then the market begins to fall. As the months roll on, it continues to fall. After a year it is still falling. By now your account is down 20%. Is the end in sight or will it continue falling? Even though you are a long term investor and believe the market will ultimately recover, this has to hurt! How would you feel to see your account balance slowly being reduced by $10,000 over that period and not know how much farther it might fall. Reading your quarterly statements will become depressing, and seeing your account balance drop, even though you are still contributing, will **really** be depressing! Are you tempted to move some or all of your money to safer options to preserve what's left? It's gut check time for your risk tolerance.

While this scenario is distressing, it does happen and the long term investor doesn't panic. These events are often considered buying opportunities by many and a chance to re-evaluate the current market trends and reallocate your investments. When the market is down your contributions buy more shares for your account. And when the market recovers, those shares appreciate even more than the older shares purchased at a higher price. Even though it is depressing to endure market downturns, many advisors suggest you may wish to re-allocate some of your assets, but basically hang in there. Stocks are on sale.

As you near retirement, it is natural to become more cautious. After all, you have spent all those years building your account. You don't want to take a large sudden loss just before time to begin cashing in! Many experts recommend reallocating more of your account to more conservative investments as time progresses.

Paper loss vs. real loss. It is important to understand the difference between a paper loss and a real loss to your portfolio. Let's say you are in a market downturn and your account has been reduced over a short time by 8%. Have you lost 8%? Maybe, or maybe not. If you withdraw money during the downturn you will have a real loss. The amount withdrawn will not have a chance to recover when the market rebounds. If you leave the money in the account, it has a chance to recover. And if it recovers over time, that 8% downturn will have simply been a temporary paper loss. This reinforces the fact that most investors become more conservative as the time for withdrawal approaches, not wanting to take a sudden loss at a time when they need to withdraw from their account.

Managing Your Account

Establish online access. Your provider should allow web access to your account. You will need to establish a login name and password, and you can then monitor the progress of your investments. If you have trouble gaining access, contact your Plan Administrator.

Review your allocation periodically. Examine how your money is invested at least once per year to see if it is still appropriate. You may wish to reconsider investment choices and percentage allocations as you get older, your risk tolerance changes, or if you believe fundamental market changes are occurring. It is tempting to reallocate and move money into those funds that were hot last year. Many experts recommend not chasing last year's big performers. Often they cannot duplicate those gains the following year. Instead, maintain a long term diversified outlook. Make small modifications once or twice a year if required. Remember the story of the Hare and the Tortoise?

Check your withholding and account deposits. Examine your pay stubs and be sure the correct amount is being withheld each pay period. Go online periodically and check your account to verify deposits are being made within a reasonable period. Contact your Plan Administrator if you feel deposits are not accurate or unreasonably delayed.

> *Insight* *Over a two year period an agency missed deposits totaling several hundred dollars. The traveler insisted they review the situation. The agency quickly found the error and corrected the account. But it never would have happened if the traveler hadn't checked the account and forced the issue. Mistakes happen. Be sure to verify the agency's deposits.*

Learn more about investing and the Stock Market. Spend an hour or so each week expanding your knowledge of investing. You can use any search engine to find a wealth of information on the web. Many investment firms such as Vanguard, Fidelity, etc., have excellent reference material. Tune into financial news programs such as CNBC to help gain a broad market perspective. Your expanded knowledge will allow you to track market trends and help you make informed decisions as economic conditions change.

Consolidating Old Accounts

You may accumulate several 401(k) accounts as you change agencies, and it can be difficult to keep track of your investments. If you float between several agencies, leave your 401(k) open at each. It's a hassle to track, but it keeps those accounts available if you accept another assignment with that agency.

If you will not be returning to an agency, consider rolling over your 401(k) to an IRA. IRA's often have more investment options. You can open a brokerage account to encompass all your mutual funds that also allows you to purchase individual stocks.

Be sure to do an "institution to institution" rollover. Your current 401(k) administrator transfers your money directly to the new investment company handling the IRA. No money passes through your hands. This avoids the possibility of any tax issues and avoids the automatic 20% tax withholding. Usually there is no charge for this rollover service but occasionally a 401(k) provider will charge a small liquidation fee.

If you have a Roth 401(k) transfer it to a Roth IRA to maintain your tax-free status. If you have a Traditional 401(k) consider transferring it to a Roth IRA. You will have to pay taxes on the money that year but subsequent growth will be tax free. The other choice is to transfer it to a Traditional IRA and continue to defer taxes until the money is ultimately withdrawn. You can have a Traditional IRA and a Roth IRA at the same time. It's not an either-or situation.

Notes

Notes

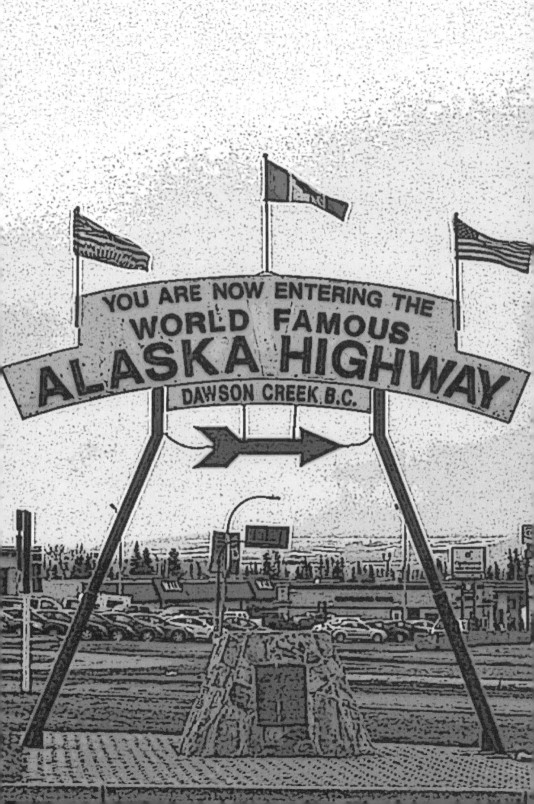

International Traveling

*I need to learn a foreign language. My family has
suggested English as a good starting point.*

Whether you are a U.S. citizen wishing to travel abroad or a foreigner wishing to work in the U.S., international travel can be an exciting (and challenging) way to expand your universe.

Foreign Healthcare Workers Entering the U.S.

America has always been the Land of Opportunity. It is said that almost everyone in America is an immigrant either directly or through ancestry. There is even speculation that Native Americans may have migrated to North America via a land bridge connecting Siberia and Alaska over ten thousand years ago.

The national nursing shortage has increased the interest in foreign healthcare workers entering the U.S. labor market. Many feel foreign workers can at least ease the shortage. However, given the diversity of educational standards throughout the world, there is concern by some regarding the quality of the healthcare and the communication skill of foreign workers.

As with other immigrants, foreign healthcare workers seeking em-ployment in the U.S. must obtain a visa to enter the country. They must also have the appropriate licensure for their specialty.

Fortunately there are many travel agencies that focus on placement of foreign healthcare workers in the U.S. Some are based in the U.S. and many others are abroad. They can explain the immigration pro-cess and will be aware of any recent changes in immigration law, entry procedures, and fees. You may wish to use the web and search strings such as "international nursing agencies" or "foreign nurse re-cruitment" to find agencies placing foreign healthcare workers in the U.S. Also, you may wish to visit web sites such as www.travelnurse-toolbox.com and www.nursetraveler.org for information on interna-tional traveling.

U.S. immigration law requires foreign healthcare workers, other than physicians, to complete a screening program to qualify for an occupa-tional visa. This process is known as a "visa screen". Applicants who successfully complete the process receive a visa screen certificate which is then used as part of the visa application.

The Commission on Graduates of Foreign Nursing Schools (CGFNS) offers this screening program. CGFNS created a division called the International Commission on Healthcare Professions (ICHP) to ad-minister their program called "VisaScreen". The VisaScreen program consists of an educational analysis, licensure validation, an English language proficiency evaluation, and an exam of nursing knowl-edge.

Educational review. This helps insure the applicant's education meets the requirements for the specialty to be practiced in the U.S. and is comparable to a U.S. graduate seeking licensure.

The applicant must have:

* Successfully completed a senior secondary education separate from their professional education.

* Graduated from a professional healthcare program of at least two years and completed a minimum number of hours in clinical and theoretical areas. The program must be approved by the U.S. Government. Also, physical therapists must include a written summary of their supervised clinical experience.

Licensure review. Evaluates the initial, current, and past licenses to insure the applicant has completed all requirements and there are no encumbrances.

English language proficiency assessment. Confirms the applicant has the required competency in written and oral English. Currently applicants have two choices to fulfill this requirement:

* The Test of English as a Foreign Language (TOEFL), Test of Spoken English (TSE) and Test of Written English (TWE).
                          Or

* The Michigan English Language Assessment Battery (MELAB) parts 1-4. This includes an oral interview and speaking test.

Some applicants are exempt from the language proficiency assessment. Their professional education must have been in Australia, Canada (excluding Quebec), Ireland, New Zealand, United Kingdom, or the U.S. The language of instruction and the textbooks must have been in English.

TN status. The North American Free Trade Agreement (NAFTA) created a special category of visa called TN status (**T**reaty **N**AFTA). This is an employment-based, temporary work visa for Canadian and Mexican citizens only. The foreign applicant must have an employer sponsor, be eligible to work in the U.S. under one of the approved categories, and must have the qualifying education, experience, license, and required credentials. It is good for one year but can be renewed each year indefinitely. The procedure for entry by Mexican citizens is slightly different than for Canadians. Your agency should be familiar with the process and documents required, and the procedure to leave and re-enter the U.S. Here are the eligible NAFTA medical and allied health professional specialties, along with their requirements:

Dentist
D.D.S., D.M.D., Doctor en Odontologia or Doctor en Cirugia Dental; or state/provincial license

Dietitian
Baccalaureate or Licenciatura Degree; or state/provincial license

Medical Laboratory Technologist (Canada)
Medical Technologist (Mexico and the United States)
Baccalaureate or Licenciatura Degree; or Post-Secondary Diploma or Post-Secondary Certificate, and three years experience

Nutritionist
Baccalaureate or Licenciatura Degree

Occupational Therapist
Baccalaureate or Licenciatura Degree; or state/provincial license

Pharmacist
Baccalaureate or Licenciatura Degree; or state/provincial license

Physician (teaching or research only)
M.D. or Doctor en Medicina; or state/provincial license

Physiotherapist
Physical Therapist
Baccalaureate or Licenciatura Degree; or state/provincial license

Psychologist
State/provincial license; or Licenciatura Degree

Recreational Therapist
Baccalaureate or Licenciatura Degree

Registered Nurse
State/provincial license; or Licenciatura Degree

Veterinarian
D.V.M., D.M.V. or Doctor en Veterinaria; or state/provincial license

H-1B visa. If you are not eligible for TN status, it may be possible to enter the U.S. under an H-1B visa. This is also an employment-based visa category for temporary workers. An employer offers the foreigner a job and submits the visa application. If approved, the applicant can enter the U.S. and work for that employer. Unlike TN status, nurses are not specifically listed as eligible for an H-1B visa, and there are yearly quota restrictions. Your agency can determine if you can qualify for an H-1B visa. You should also be aware of the procedures to leave and re-enter the U.S., change employers if necessary, the rules for bringing family members to the U.S., etc.

In 2002, the Immigration and Naturalization Service issued a memorandum clarifying when a registered nurse will be eligible for an H-1B work visa. The memorandum, HQISD 70/6.2.8-P dated November 27, 2002, was issued by the Office of Field Operations. The memo-

randum lists several healthcare specialties that may be eligible for
H-1B status. There is also a stipulation allowing an applicant to substitute experience for the required formal degree. Quoting from the
memorandum:

> "In determining degree equivalencies, the Service uses a
> formula that requires the beneficiary to have three years
> of specialized training and/or work experience for each
> year of college-level training that the beneficiary is lack-
> ing."

The INS will evaluate and accept the training and/or experience on a
case-by-case basis. The clarification memo will help insure a consis-
tent review policy by the INS. The four page memorandum is available on the web. You can locate it by entering a search string such as
"INS memo 27 Nov 2002".

The Green Card. If you plan to pursue U.S. citizenship, the green
card is a must. This is a permanent visa to the U.S. Normally it is
good for ten years at which time it will have to be re-validated. It
gives the legal right to work in the U.S. and grants permanent resident status. Within certain limits, it allows the holder to leave and
return to the U.S. while still maintaining citizenship in their original
country. You can usually apply for citizenship after you have your
Green Card for five years.

U.S. Citizens Working Abroad

For U.S. healthcare workers the allure of traveling can extend to countries abroad. Many travelers would love to live and work overseas,
and some foreign countries are increasingly recruiting U.S. healthcare
workers. The most popular destinations seem to be English speaking
countries such as the U.K., Australia, and New Zealand. As you might
expect, traveling overseas can be much different. In general the pay
is less. Travelers report you can expect to make somewhere in the

upper $30,000 to the upper $40,000 per year. Depending on location and specialty you may receive close to $50,000 per year.

You will have to be patient. Researching agencies that can place you overseas and submitting the proper paper work can take many months.

You will also need to be aware of tax issues associated with working abroad. Tax treaties exist between many countries and, of course, the tax laws within each country differ. Your agency and tax advisor should be able to clarify this issue. I recommend downloading the latest copy of IRS Publication 54 *"Tax Guide for U.S. Citizens and Resident Aliens Abroad".* It's available from www.irs.gov, or enter "IRS publication 54" into your search engine to find a copy. In tax year 2008 earned income up to $87,600 was excluded from U.S. taxation if you qualified. The maximum is adjusted annually for inflation so be sure and check the latest edition. The rules for qualifying are also defined in Publication 54. Here's a quote from the 2008 edition:

> "To claim the foreign earned income exclusion, the foreign housing exclusion, or the foreign housing deduction, you must meet all three of the following requirements.
>
> 1. Your tax home must be in a foreign country.
> 2. You must have foreign earned income.
> 3. You must be either:
>   a. A U.S. citizen who is a bona fide resident of a foreign country or countries for an uninterrupted period that includes an entire tax year.
>   b. A U.S. resident alien who is a citizen or national of a country with which the United States has an income tax treaty in effect and who is a bona fide resident of a foreign country or countries for an uninterrupted period that includes an entire tax year, or
>   c. A U.S. citizen or a U.S. resident alien who is physically present in a foreign country or countries for at least 330 full days during any period of 12 consecutive months."

As indicated, you may also qualify for a foreign housing exclusion or deduction.

Be aware that you may have a tax liability in the country you are working. IRS Publication 54 has a listing of the countries with which the U.S. has a tax treaty and also describes the procedure for acquiring a copy of the treaty. Your agency should have a good idea of tax liabilities in the various countries with which they have dealt.

Traveling abroad can be fun and rewarding but you need to have a good idea of what to expect. Be sure you understand all the details of working abroad including your housing, benefits, working conditions, and tax issues. Situations overseas can differ greatly from what you have encountered in the U.S. While in a foreign country you are subject to their laws and must adhere to the local social mores. Some countries, such as those in the Middle East, have significant cultural differences. This can be restrictive and challenging.

Notes

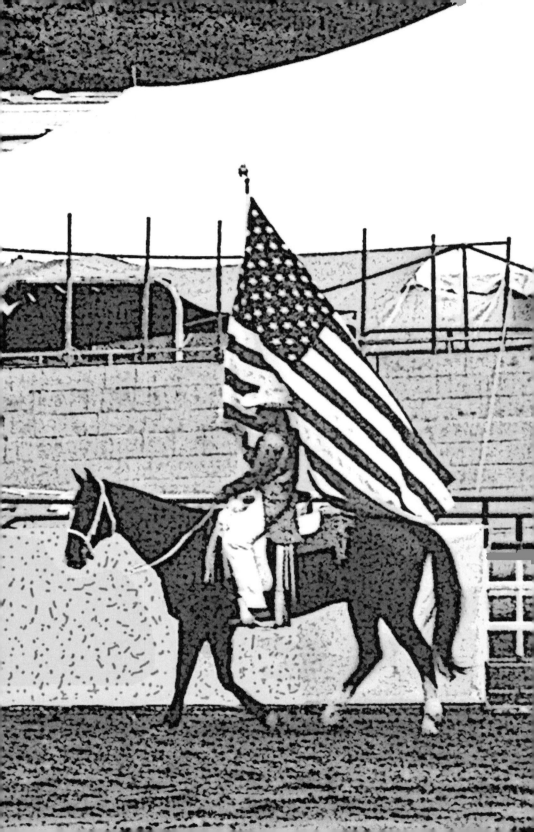

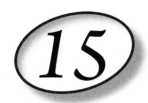

Miscellaneous Issues

"Miscellaneous" is a rather pompous sounding word used when you have no idea what you have or where it goes.

*A*fter traveling for awhile you begin to settle into a certain comfort zone. You have probably found several agencies you can work with. They in turn have developed a comfort level when dealing with you. They know your personality, talents, and needs. They know they can count on you to produce quality healthcare at each assignment. This makes both you and the agency look good and increases your marketability. All this leads to . . .

Establishing a Basis for Trust

This basis for trust allows both the traveler and the agency to benefit. You have good pay and great assignments. Negotiations become easier once the two parties know what to expect from each other. The agency may also be willing to pay for smaller costs that occasionally occur and are not specifically included in the contract. If you are a valuable traveler, they want to keep you onboard and happy. Here are a couple of examples of the value of a trusted relationship:

❊ A traveler was ill and had to miss two shifts. She called her agency and asked that her tax-exempt items not be reduced. The agency knew she was a good worker and would not miss unless absolutely necessary. She did not receive wages for the two shifts but her tax-free items, including housing and M&IE, were not reduced.

❊ A traveler had worked for an agency for awhile but had taken an assignment with another to be close to relatives. The assignment turned out to be a nightmare and the traveler felt her license was in jeopardy. She called her original agency to see if anything could be done. The agency knew she was a valuable worker. They bought out the problem contract and placed the traveler in a much better assignment.

Agencies know how the game is played. Even though you often develop personal relationships with your recruiters the bottom line is that it is still a business. Make it clear to each of your recruiters that you will give them a fair chance to compete for your service. Treat them fairly . . . just like you want to be treated.

If you have difficulty with an agency or recruiter, try to leave on good terms. The long road of traveling has many twists and turns. Although you may be angry at the moment, a profitable opportunity may arise with that agency or recruiter later. Try not to burn any bridges.

Employment Testing

Facilities have the responsibility to insure their healthcare workers are experienced, qualified, and competent. Some use testing as a way to assess the ability of both permanent and temporary personnel.

Some facilities use the **P**erformance **B**ased **D**evelopment **S**ystem (**PBDS**) developed by Performance Management Services, Inc. (http://www.pmsi-pbds.com/). It is a customized competency assessment used to evaluate the ability of hospital personnel to do their job. The test is specially designed for the needs of each facility and usually takes four to six hours to complete. The format varies but consists mostly of video segments presenting various scenarios. The healthcare worker then answers questions regarding what they have observed.

A few facilities apparently use the test as employment criteria. If you fail the test your contract may be cancelled. Other facilities apparently use it only to identify areas where additional orientation or education may be helpful. Some travelers do not interview with facilities that require the test. Even some who have taken and passed the test say they will not take it again.

Another test is the **B**asic **K**nowledge **A**ssessment **T**ool (**BKAT**) and is related to critical care nursing. The tests are paper and pencil with multiple choice and fill-in the blank questions. For a list of the latest modules and a description of each, you can visit http://nursing.cua.edu/research/. As with PBDS, some travelers choose not to interview with facilities that require it.

When interviewing for an assignment, be sure to ask if the facility requires employment testing. If so, ask what test and module you will have to take . . . and be sure you understand how the results will be used.

Working Strikes

Some facilities are unionized. Occasionally a union feels the need to strike to receive the increase in pay and benefits they feel they deserve. When this happens supervisors and other staff attempt to fill in the gap, and the facility may hire travelers or other temporary personnel to take the place of the striking workers.

There is a difference of opinion when it comes to working strikes. Some travelers refuse to cross the picket line feeling they may prolong the strike by reducing the pressure on management to settle. They may also feel a certain loyalty to their fellow healthcare professionals. Other travelers feel it is alright to take the place of striking workers. They feel it is necessary to insure quality patient care while negotiations proceed.

A few agencies specialize in providing travelers for strikes. If a strike appears eminent, the facility may ask an agency to provide healthcare workers. They are usually housed in a nearby motel awaiting the call to go to work. It's possible for them to remain there from several days to perhaps a couple of weeks, or more. If the strike is called they are transported to the facility to begin work. For personal safety reasons they may have to live at the facility for the duration of the strike. If the strike is cancelled they go home, all the while being paid well. If you wish to participate in a strike assignment, you may want to visit http://www.scab.org.

Breaking Your Contract

Your contract is a legally binding document for both you and your agency. It should not be taken lightly. You should make every effort to complete your assignment. If you have a bad experience with the facility or the agency, move on after the contract is completed. Being lonely, homesick, or deciding you are not happy with the pay and benefit package are not good reasons to leave an assignment. However there are times when breaking your contract could be appropriate.

Personal reasons. Serious injury and illness can happen anytime to you or a member of your immediate family. Discuss the situation with your recruiter and your supervisor if you feel you have documented circumstances that make it difficult to fulfill your contract. Your agency may be able to send another traveler to finish the assignment, or the facility may be able to work around your absence if it is not too prolonged.

Professional reasons. Travelers sometimes complain of unsafe working conditions. You may be put in situations where you feel patient safety is at risk. Too many patients or too many very sick patients can make it difficult to give the quality care required.

Occasionally you may find a coworker's actions intimidating and perhaps even threatening. You do not have to endure harassment.

The facility may violate the letter or spirit of the contract. Excessive float beyond the agreement, and float to areas where you are not fully qualified are a couple of complaints. Excessive shift cancellation can also occur, which could substantially reduce your income.

Talk to your recruiter and your supervisor if these or other problems occur. If the situation cannot be resolved your agency should consider canceling the assignment. Remember, in some cases your license could be at stake! There may be some financial penalties for leaving a contract early. This usually involves your housing. Most agencies will work to minimize the impact and often allow you to slowly repay the amount owed on your next assignment.

Contracts have also been cancelled for unsafe or unavailable housing. Your agency should provide good, safe housing. Granted in some areas this can be a challenge. If you really feel unsafe and your agency cannot or will not provide safe housing, perhaps you should consider moving on.

You should notify the facility and agency in writing as to why you are terminating your contract. Be sure to include any documentation available.

Are Foreign Nurses a Threat?

The national nursing shortage has created increased opportunities for foreign nurses and other healthcare workers to work in the U.S. The question arises as to whether patient care might be jeopardized by foreign workers if they are not fully qualified. The agencies and facilities have the obligation to screen foreign workers thoroughly to be sure they are capable of performing to U.S. healthcare standards. The visa screen process also helps assure foreign workers are qualified. While facilities and staff will probably welcome the help of foreign nurses, they don't have time to train the foreign worker on skills and knowledge they should already possess. Staff members are sometimes concerned that the communication skills of some foreign workers are not as good as they need to be. For example, some feel this could present problems during shift change report when critical information is exchanged.

The question also arises as to whether current wage levels may be threatened by foreign workers. While researching information for this book I discovered an agency indicating they could provide H-1B visa healthcare workers at a lower wage than travel nurses but who could provide continuity of patient care. If it's possible to recruit qualified foreign healthcare workers for less, is your job in jeopardy? I'll leave it for you to decide.

Special California Issues

There are a couple of special issues associated with working in California. One deals with overtime, the other with taxes.

There is sometimes a misunderstanding about overtime in California. In most other states, overtime is paid only after 40 hours have been worked per week. If you work 42 hours in a week you will receive two hours in overtime pay. If you work 10 hours one day, 12 hours the next but don't exceed 40 hours per week, you usually will not receive overtime pay.

California has a "daily overtime" law. The rate is time and one half after 8 hours and double time after 12. If you work 10 hours one day, 12 hours the next but don't exceed 40 hours per week you should still receive overtime pay for the six hours you worked beyond your eight hour shift.

However, there is an exception to the law. By a two-thirds vote the facility may adopt an "alternative work week" where overtime is paid differently than specified in the daily overtime law. An example would be a schedule consisting of four 10 hour shifts. The facility may then pay its employees regular time for those hours. Any time over 40 would be at the overtime rate. The bottom line is if you accept an assignment in California you should be paid overtime under the same scenario as the permanent staff at that facility. And hopefully it will be under the daily overtime law.

Some agencies claim to be exempt from this special law because they are located outside the state. My understanding is if they conduct business in California they must pay overtime to their travelers at the same rate the facility pays its own staff regardless of their corporate location. Be sure to clarify the overtime issue with your agency prior to accepting a California assignment.

The second special issue deals with tax residency. The requirements to determine state residency for tax purposes varies per state. According to The State of California Franchise Tax Board, FTB Publication 1031, *Guidelines for Determining Resident Status – 2007,* California may consider you a full time resident after only nine months.

If you have a temporary assignment in California and have a permanent tax home in another state, you should have little difficulty proving you are "temporary or transitory" even if you stay longer than nine months. But be sure to consider this when accepting California assignments and signing contract extensions. If this situation applies to you, download the latest version of FTB Publication 1031 from http://www.ftb.ca.gov/, and check the wording. Your tax advisor may have an opinion on this as well.

Your Recruiter – Friend or Foe?

Tune into any discussion forum and you will probably read horror stories from travelers regarding their agency or recruiter. From the writer's stand point they are dealing with some kind of inflexible, foul, fire-breathing beast. And of course the traveler is never at fault!

While some agencies are better than others, and "issues" may arise, there are many excellent agencies with good recruiters. They are certainly in business to make a profit. And that profit comes from the hard work of those under contract. But most realize they must treat their travelers well to stay in business. By talking to other travelers and doing your research you can avoid problem agencies and recruiters.

Some travelers feel if the agency makes a dime, it's a dime they should have. We have never felt that way. We certainly do not want them to overly enrich themselves at our expense but we want them to make a decent living, just as we expect. They need to buy a house, send their kids to college, and generally prosper. Frankly, I want our recruiters to be in a good mood when they are getting our next assignment.

We have traveled for over seven years with good pay and good assignments. We have seen much of America and have done things we never thought possible. Did we squeeze every nickel from each assignment? I'm sure we left many on the table. But given our experience, I believe your recruiter is your friend.

The Future of Traveling

I was up in the attic the other day and found my old crystal ball. Let's dust it off and do a little gazing.

The national nursing shortage. The shortage of quality healthcare workers will continue well into the future. While nursing schools are continuing to graduate as many as they can as quickly as they can, the population is aging at a faster pace. Any field dealing with geriatrics should experience increasing, even explosive needs for healthcare workers. You may notice increased use of foreign nurses to help ease the shortage.

Nurse Licensure Compact. The trend toward a national license will accelerate. Every few years one or two states join. When the compact reaches beyond the midpoint the rest of the states will begin to "wake up" to the benefits and join at an increasing rate.

Agency consolidation. It astounds me that well over 200 U.S. agencies are in the business of placing travelers. Agencies pop up and others go out of business regularly. Keeping an accurate, current list is very difficult. The trend toward JCAHO certification will make it harder for new agencies to get started. Some smaller agencies may need to merge with larger ones to survive. I don't expect it to boil down to just a few super agencies, but the number of agencies may be reduced by half in the next ten to twenty years.

Hospital associations. The hospital associations will continue to exist but may have less impact. Legal actions may reduce their effectiveness (Example: United States of America and the State of Arizona v. Arizona Hospital and Healthcare Association and AzHHA Service Corporation, Case No. CV07-1030-PHX, filed May 22, 2007). If the nursing shortage continues or worsens, or if enough travelers avoid those areas, facilities may feel the need to bypass the associations in order to attract qualified employees, both permanent staff and travelers.

Technological advances. Advances in diagnostics and testing will continue. Body scans and other imaging will detect problems sooner and will allow increased treatment by non-interventional methods. This could reduce the need for surgical intervention and may ultimately have an impact on the workload in some of the special procedures areas. Automation of nursing notes and other documentation will continue. Eventually it may be difficult to find a pencil or pen at the nursing station!

Health insurance. Don't expect significant changes in the health insurance system. No major changes are likely to happen for many years, if ever. Every election cycle we hear the same old cry for change. But I expect Congress will continue to have difficulty reaching a consensus. Only band-aid proposals have a chance. The good news is that travelers will continue to be needed and can expect to be well paid for a long time to come.

Notes

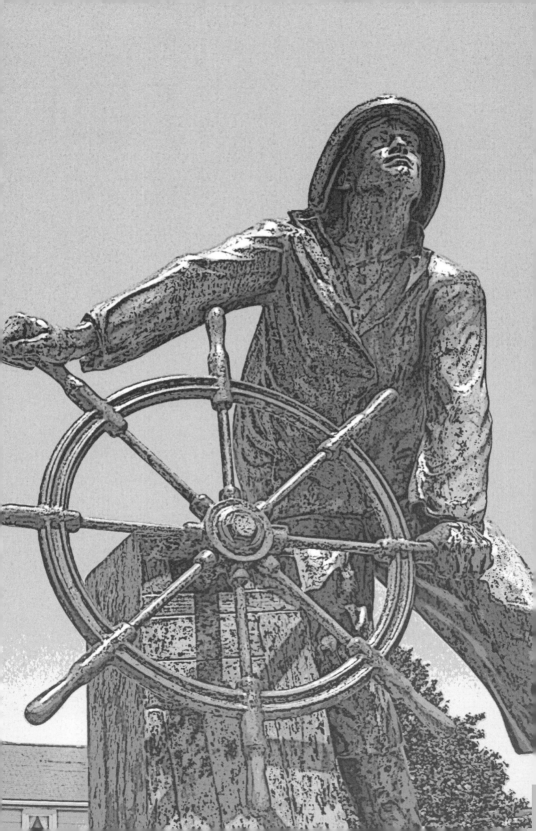

16

The Darker Side of Traveling

What passes for normal may only be an acceptable form of chaos.

*I*f you are a seasoned traveler, you have no doubt noticed some interesting things when dealing with facilities, staffing agencies, permanent staffers, and other travelers. Let's start with . . .

The Facility

By and large the facilities need help. Most appreciate travelers and treat them well. However some facilities have issues. Here are some circumstances you may have encountered either as a traveler or a permanent staffer:

The clueless manager. You wonder why some supervisors and managers are even there. Some almost seem to be hiding! Between being off and shutting themselves in their office, they are seldom visible and seem to have little interest in what is happening in their area. Often one or more permanent staffers are left to run the unit. However, they may not have the authority to make certain decisions at the spur of the moment as needed. This may cause occasional work flow chaos and generate hard feelings in the unit. And as a traveler you could be "the odd man out".

The egomaniac staffer. As a traveler you will have to prove your-self at each new assignment. No matter that you have 10 years of ex-perience in your specialty. Granted you need to be flexible, and they need to know your skills. But sometimes you run into a permanent staffer who thinks they are God's gift to medicine. And Heaven help you if they have to check you off on certain procedures!

Staff resentment. There may be resentment by some permanent staffers toward travelers. Frankly, I suspect many are jealous of the freedom and extra pay of the traveler. Perhaps the staffer feels trapped or frustrated in their situation. In any case, you do not have to endure harassment.

> **Insight** *A traveler was just finishing their lunch break in the caf-eteria when a permanent staffer asked for their advice regarding a patient. The conversation took awhile and when the traveler returned to the unit another permanent staffer remarked, "Well, looks like travelers can take as much lunch time as they want!"*

The unit is overstaffed. A facility sometimes hires travelers even though they are staffed appropriately. The management may want to keep their permanent staffers as happy as possible to keep them onboard. Travelers can not only ease the existing work load but allow the permanent staff to "cruise" during the day and focus on overtime to increase their pay.

Taking all the call. There always seems to be one or two permanent staffers that want to take everyone's call. They use it to augment their regular salary. Many travelers appreciate less call and don't mind. You may have problems if you are counting on call or call back pay as extra income. Oh, sure, you might get some call: on a three day weekend when everyone wants to be off!

Manipulating the workload to increase overtime. At a special procedures unit the permanent staff dragged their feet during the morning. This pushed afternoon cases into overtime. The travelers left at the end of their shift. The permanent staff stayed and completed the cases on overtime.

Unfair workload. Travelers may be given the tougher cases, and be the first to float to other units.

Using travelers PRN. You may have a clause in your contract saying the facility has the right to reschedule your shifts. Some facilities abuse this by excessive rescheduling and sometimes canceling shifts. This is where the contract is important. You should have a clause guaranteeing your hours and one stating your housing, daily living allowance, etc., will not be reduced for cancelled shifts. Also, if cancelled shifts become a problem, your recruiter should call the facility and insist they live up to the spirit and terms of the contract.

The Traveler

By far the overwhelming majority of travelers are competent, qualified, and well motivated. However, a few have issues:

The "painful" traveler. We mentioned earlier why some become travelers. They travel for adventure, extra money, etc. There's another reason some become travelers: they have trouble holding down a permanent job. Most seem to have the necessary skills for their specialty but may not work well with the doctors and permanent staff. And their attitude toward patients may need some adjustment. By the time the facility realizes what a pain they are, they are usually well into the contract. The facility often endures their antics and lets them complete the assignment. Why? They need help. Even if that help is a pain! Sometimes the facility is so desperate for help they are even willing to extend the contract of a problem traveler.

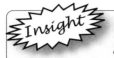 *We have seen one traveler's contract cancelled prior to completion. The facility simply could not tolerate their antics any longer.*

Fraudulently accepting a travel advance. Your agency will probably not give you a travel advance to get to your assignment. They may buy your plane ticket but will seldom give you cash up front. You have to claim it on your first time sheet. Wonder why? Stories have circulated in the past about travelers signing contracts, receiving the advance, and then not reporting to work. The agency then has to try to get their money back!

Abusing time off. We have mentioned several times that your tax-free payments will be prorated for working less than your full weekly schedule. This seems rather harsh. If you are sick for a day or two what's the big deal? Your agency can afford the few extra bucks for those days. The problem is that some travelers abuse the practice, taking unnecessary and excessive time off while under contract. Keep in mind the agency can only receive payment from the facility for hours worked, and excessive absence can be a drain on the agency's bottom line for that assignment.

Substance abuse issues. Some healthcare workers (not just travelers) have at least periodic problems passing a drug screen. They work as allowed.

The Agency

Any agency worth its salt will offer their travelers a decent assignment package with good pay, housing, and benefits. They know where their bread is buttered. Without the traveler, many would be out of business. However, all agencies are not "created equal". Here are some issues that may be encountered:

Bill rate secrecy. Agencies will normally not reveal the exact bill rate for a particular job. This is part of their negotiation strategy. They may give you a range for the general area you are in, say the Northeast. This prevents you from knowing exactly how much profit they are making at your expense. They may not reveal other items as well, such as the exact cost of housing.

Bait and switch. An agency may market a highly qualified candidate to a facility knowing the traveler has no intention of accepting the assignment. The agency strings the facility along until close to the assignment start date then offers another traveler at the last minute claiming the original traveler declined the assignment. The facility probably accepts the substitute rather than start the search over again and wasting more time. And the agency fills the opening rather than a competitor.

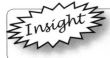

If your agency asks you to interview for an assignment for which you have no interest, you may be participating in some form of bait and switch.

Placing difficult travelers. As mentioned, some travelers are consistently hard to work with. They make themselves and the agency look bad. Why do agencies continue to place them? Simple: there are big bucks at stake. Every 13 week contract is money in their pocket. The agency can rationalize that this time may be different. Maybe this time the traveler will find a group they can gel with. Eventually the agency may decide to stop offering assignments to a problem traveler. By the way, it's easy for an agency to terminate its relationship with a traveler. Each time the traveler calls, the agency "doesn't have any openings in your specialty right now".

Phantom benefits. Agencies will sometimes offer a benefit and then make it difficult for the traveler to qualify. Paid time off is sometimes an example. For instance an agency may offer to give you one week of pay after working, say, 1920 hours. However, they may state that those hours must be regular hours (overtime does not count) and must be accumulated in a single calendar year. This means you would have to work almost continuously from sometime in January well into December. While some travelers may qualify, many change assignments and agencies fairly often. Travelers also tend to take time off throughout the year, perhaps a week or two between assignments and some for the Holiday period. Given this lifestyle, some travelers may have difficulty qualifying for this benefit.

Occasionally you may find an agency that offers a 401(k) plan but makes you wait up to one year to enroll. Again, this may be a dubious benefit given the lifestyle of some travelers.

Cold calling. Be aware that some states sell your license data. This can lead to mail and phone calls from agencies you have never dealt with and perhaps have never even heard of.

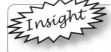 *We always list our permanent home phone number on all license applications and check for messages remotely. This helps protect our cell phone numbers.*

Cold calling is not all bad. It gives you an opportunity to learn more about an agency and their offerings. You could actually benefit from the practice. If you receive a cold call and the recruiter gives you enough details of an assignment that sounds interesting, you can call your recruiter to see if they can get you there. Some travelers report receiving cold calls while at work. This is considered unethical.

Your agency goes out of business. There have been reports of agencies going out of business abruptly and stranding their travelers on assignment. Hopefully there is at least one other agency working with the facility that can hire the travelers and keep them in place for the duration of their contract. If not, the traveler may ask another agency to step in and pick up the contract. The facility may be willing to freeze payments to the defunct agency to attempt to help the travelers recoup their earnings. If this happens to you, follow up on any pay items owed to you. Also, be sure to check the status of those items your agency was responsible for such as your housing, 401(k) deposits to your account, insurance issues, taxes withheld, etc.

The disappearing recruiter. You just love your recruiter. They have found you good assignments with good pay and stays in touch. Things are going great. Then one day you call and are told your recruiter no longer works there. What happened? You thought you had a great relationship and they left without even a goodbye phone call. That was rude!

Occasionally recruiters change agencies. Sometimes they open a competing agency. Lawsuits have been filed against recruiters for "stealing" travelers when they left their agency. To avoid this problem the recruiter usually will not contact their old travelers first. They depend on the traveler to find them and establish first contact. This way the recruiter cannot be accused of stealing the traveler. If you wish to contact your former recruiter, hopefully you have their cell phone number. If not, they may be difficult to locate. There have even been posts on discussion forums from travelers trying to find a former recruiter. Some feel this is a restraint of trade. After all, why should you have to go on a scavenger hunt to find your old business connection.

Notes

Notes

A Final Word

So what do you think? Is traveling right for you? As you see there are a lot of things involved and much to consider.

I hope you have found this book interesting and informative. Again, no one source of information can be considered as a complete treatment of the subject. Indeed several topics, such as taxes, investing, negotiating, and independent contracting, could easily comprise separate publications. By talking to travelers, consulting other publications, and using the extensive information on the web, you can continue to expand your knowledge and tailor the information to fit your individual situation and needs.

We have found traveling fun and rewarding. It has allowed us to see and do things we could have only imagined. We have been off for extended periods when we wanted and still made a good living. Will we travel forever? Of course not. But as long as we enjoy it and can do the things we want, why not!

And who knows, maybe we'll see you on the road!

Barry Padgett

P.S. If you have an interesting experience as a traveler and would like to share it in a revision of the book, please send it to the address below. Please include a phone number or e-mail address so I can contact you if needed. Your suggestions and comments will also be appreciated. Thanks!

> Barry Padgett
> c/o Buffalo Nickel Publishing LLC
> PO Box 850458
> Mobile, Alabama 36685-0458

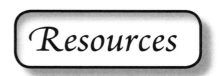
Resources

Here are some of the resources you may find useful as a traveler:

Airlines

Alaska Air www.alaskaair.com

Continental www.continental.com

Delta www.delta.com

Frontier www.frontierairlines.com

JetBlue www.jetblue.com

Midwest www.midwestairlines.com

Skywest www.skywest.com

Southwest www.southwest.com

United www.united.com

US Airways/America West www.usairways.com

Car rental

Alamo www.alamo.com

Avis www.avis.com

Budget www.budget.com

Enterprise www.enterprise.com

Hertz www.hertz.com

National www.nationalcar.com

Thrifty www.thrifty.com

Federal Agencies and Acts

COBRA www.dol.gov/dol/topic/health-plans/cobra.htm

GSA www.gsa.gov

HIPAA Summary: www.hhs.gov/ocr/privacysummary.pdf

IRS www.irs.gov

OSHA www.osha.gov

GPS navigation
Garmin www.garmin.com
Magellan www.magellan.com
Mio www.mio.com
Tomtom www.TomTom.com

IRS publications (from www.irs.gov)
54 - Tax Guide for U.S. Citizens and Resident Aliens Abroad
463 - Travel, Entertainment, Gift, and Car Expenses
1542 - Per Diem Rates (For Travel Within the Continental
    United States

Motel locations and evaluations
American Automobile Association TourBooks www.aaa.com

Online travel agencies
Cheap tickets www.cheaptickets.com
Expedia www.expedia.com
Travelocity www.travelocity.com

Road map and atlas publications
American Automobile Association www.aaa.com
American Map www.americanmap.com
Rand McNally www.randmcnally.com

Road atlas software
Rand McNally www.randmcnally.com

Roadside assistance programs
American Automobile Association www.aaa.com
Your auto insurance company may offer a program.
Your auto manufacturer may offer a program.

RV campground directories

Trailer Life www.trailerlifedirectory.com
Woodall's www.woodalls.com

RV clubs

Camp Club USA www.campclub.com
Escapees www.escapees.com
Good Sam Club www.goodsamclub.com
Happy Camper Club www.camphalfprice.com
Passport America www.passportamerica.com
The RV Club www.rvclub.com
Thousand Trails www.Thousandtrails.com

RV services and supplies

Camping World www.campingworld.com
Local RV dealers usually offer services and supplies
Wal-Mart (supplies) www.walmart.com

Shipping services

Airborne www.airborne.com
FedEx www.FedEx.com
Purolator www.purolator.com
UPS www.ups.com
USPS www.usps.gov

Travel books

American Automobile Association TourBooks www.aaa.com
Fodor's www.fodors.com
Frommer's www.fommers.com
Insider's Guide www.insidersguide.com
Insight Guides www.insighttravelguides.com
Moon Handbooks www.moon.com

Traveling healthcare profession - general information
Boards of Nursing listings
National Council of State Boards of Nursing www.ncsbn.org

AllNursingSchools www.allnursingschools.com

Books
Highway Hypodermics: Travel Nursing 2007 by Epstein LaRue

Highway Hypodermics: Your Road Map to Travel Nursing
by Epstein LaRue

Hitting the Road: A Guide to Travel Nursing
by Shalon Kearney

Magazines
Healthcare Traveler www.healthcaretraveler.com

Travel Nursing Magazine www.travelnursingmagazine.com

Web discussion forums on www.delphiforums.com
Travel Nurses & Therapists-No Recruiting

TNT Recruiting Board

ER Nurses

Independent Nurses

Laboratory Professionals

Nurses on Wheels

OB Nurses Forum

Operating Room Travelers

Travel Nurse Housing

Travel Psych Nurses

Traveling Radiology Techs

Web sites
www.highwayhypodermics.com

www.nursetraveler.org

www.pantravelers.org

www.travelnursetoolbox.com

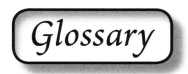

Glossary

All terms are defined within the context of this book.

401(k) *A retirement plan (Traditional or Roth) consisting of your contributions and, in some cases, matching funds from your employer.*

50 mile rule *General criteria used by some agencies to determine if tax-free reimbursements may be appropriate. Not based on IRS statute.*

apartment finder *A business used by agencies to locate appropriate housing for an assignment.*

ATM *Automated Teller Machine. Used to access cash from your bank account.*

background check *Investigation to prove your identity and detect past unlawful or unethical activity.*

benefits *Services or payments provided in addition to hourly wages.*

bill rate *The hourly rate an agency charges a facility for services of a traveler.*

BKAT *Basic Knowledge Assessment Tool. A test related to critical care nursing.*

blended rate *An average hourly wage usually calculated for 12 hour shifts. Hours over eight are paid at the overtime rate and averaged together with the eight hour shift wage.*

blind profile *A form of resume in which your name as been omitted.*

board of nursing *The state agency responsible for issuing and monitoring licenses to healthcare workers.*

bonus *Additional compensation over and above that usually expected.*

breaking a contract *Terminating a contractual agreement prior to its expiration date.*

business activity *Business relationships used by the IRS to determine your tax home.*

cafeteria plan *A special category of health plan in which you choose the coverage desired.*

call-back pay *Pay received for being called back to work after your normal shift has expired.*

car allowance *Reimbursement for expenses associated with a car while on assignment. Usually tax-free if you qualify.*

CEU *Continuing Educational Unit. Credit for each hour of instruction. Often required for licensing.*

CGFNS *Commission on Graduates of Foreign Nursing Schools. Offers the visa screen program to foreign healthcare workers attempting to enter the U.S.*

COBRA *Consolidated Omnibus Budget Reconciliation Act. Congressional legislation providing temporary health benefits to those qualified.*
cold calling *The practice of unsolicited calling of healthcare workers by agencies to inquire as to their availability for future assignments. Often based on information purchased from state licensing boards.*
combined rate *Total equivalent hourly wage including benefits.*
compact state *A member of the Nurse Licensure Compact for mutual recognition of member state licenses.*
compensation *Payment in return for work performed.*
contract *A binding agreement between two or more persons or parties.*
contract clause *An individual section of a contract dealing with a distinct concept.*
contribution limit *The yearly legal limit of money that can be added to a retirement plan.*
CONUS *Continental United States. The 48 contiguous states.*
corporate apartment *A completely furnished apartment, excluding food and personal need items.*
credit check *An inquiry into the credit worthiness of an individual or organization.*
defined benefit plan *A retirement plan providing a pension and often medical benefits. Based on an average wage and service time.*
Delphi forums *A series of discussion forums available on the web.*
deposit *Money given as a pledge of good faith in a business transaction.*
direct deposit *Money deposited electronically directly into an account.*
e-mail *Written and/or graphical information transmitted to one or more addressees via the web.*
extended stay motel *A motel offering stays of a week, month, or longer, usually at a reduced daily rate.*
facility *Any business hiring healthcare workers.*
FDIC *Federal Deposit Insurance Corporation. Insures commercial bank accounts within certain limits.*
federal tax *Tax paid to the Federal Government.*
fifth wheel *A recreational vehicle that attaches to a tow vehicle by way of a special hitch mounted in the bed of the tow vehicle.*
fill-in the blank clause *A contract clause, capable of being edited, describing a specific aspect of the assignment.*
fingerprinting *A graphic impression of the ends of the fingers used for identification purposes.*
float *Short term assignment to a unit other than your primary work area.*
furnished apartment *An apartment containing all the furniture generally expected. May or may not contain kitchen utensils.*
furnishings package *Items such as furniture, kitchen utensils, and linens provided as part of the housing.*
green card *Required documentation allowing eligibility for citizenship in the U.S.*
GSA *General Services Administration. Federal agency responsible for determining and publishing the yearly per diem rates.*

guaranteed pay *Pay received for cancelled or incomplete shifts through no fault of your own.*

H-1B visa *Allows foreign workers to enter the U.S. under certain circumstances.*

health insurance *Provides assistance in paying for medically related costs.*

HIPAA *Health Insurance Portability and Accountability Act. Sets standards to protect patient privacy.*

holiday pay *Extra compensation received for work during a holiday.*

hospital association *A group of facilities joined together to improve efficiency and reduce overall costs.*

hourly wage *Compensation for each hour of your normal shift.*

housing allowance *See "stipend".*

I-9 form *A Federal government form on which you state your legal status in the U.S.*

income tax *Tax paid yearly to the Federal and State governments based on your income.*

indefinite assignment *An assignment lasting, or expected to last, longer than one year.*

independent contractor *A traveler that assumes the duties of the agency to find and negotiate their assignment.*

international agency *A business that provides overseas facilities with healthcare workers on a temporary or permanent basis.*

investment allocation *Deciding how best to divide your money between several investments.*

investment temperament *Your tolerance for taking risk when investing.*

JCAHO *Joint Commission on Accreditation of Healthcare Organizations. Issues accreditation to qualifying facilities and staffing agencies.*

license *Document issued by the State indicating you are qualified to perform the permitted duties in that State.*

license reimbursement *Payment for costs associated with acquiring or renewing a license. Usually tax-free if you qualify.*

local agency *A business that provides facilities with healthcare workers on a temporary or permanent basis in a small area, usually in a metropolitan area.*

lodging *The portion of per diem allocated to housing.*

IRS *Internal Revenue Service. Responsible for collecting taxes for the U.S. Government.*

M&IE *The portion of per diem allocated for Meals and Incidental Expenses.*

marketability *Your qualifications and personality that enhance your ability to be selected for an assignment.*

motorhome *A recreational vehicle containing the engine within the unit.*

NAFTA *North American Free Trade Agreement. A treaty between the U.S., Canada, and Mexico to facilitate the movement of goods and services among the three countries.*

national agency *A business that provides healthcare workers on a temporary or permanent basis to facilities in areas throughout the nation.*

national nursing shortage *The situation where not enough nurses are available to fill all the openings.*

negotiations *The process by which two or more parties arrive at an agreement.*

Nurse Licensure Compact *An agreement between member States to recognize the licenses from other member States.*

OCONUS *Outside the **Con**tinental **U**nited **S**tates. U.S. States and territories outside the 48 contiguous states. Examples: Alaska and Guam.*

on-call pay *Compensation for carrying a beeper for call-back while off duty.*

online banking *The ability to perform banking transactions via the web.*

OSHA *Occupational Safety and Health Administration. Federal government agency responsible for setting standards for workplace safety.*

overtime pay *Compensation for work beyond your normal shift.*

paper loss *An unrealized loss in an investment.*

partially furnished apartment *A furnishings package for which you must provide certain additional items.*

PBDS *Performance Based Development System. A test to evaluate healthcare workers as to their knowledge in their specialty.*

per diem *Reimbursement for expenses while away from your permanent home. Usually tax-free if you qualify.*

per diem tables *Contain the maximum per diem rates for the various areas of the U.S. and overseas. Published yearly, revised as required.*

permanent home *Your permanent residence for tax purposes.*

pet deposit *Special housing deposit or costs associated with traveling with a pet.*

prn *pro re nata Latin term used in medicine to mean "as needed" or "as the situation arises". Sometimes used to describe temporary working conditions.*

profile *Similar to a resume. Contains information as to your suitability for employment. Used by agencies to present you to a facility as a candidate for an assignment*

qualifying event *Criteria allowing eligibility for a program or benefit. Example: Eligibility for COBRA.*

real loss *Removing all or part of a monetary account that has lost value.*

recreational vehicle *A mobile unit used for living and traveling purposes.*

recruiter *An agency or facility employee responsible for retaining and placing personnel.*

regional agency *Staffing agency placing travelers within a particular region of the country, such as the Northeast.*

registry *A listing of available temporary personnel maintained by a facility or staffing agency.*

risk tolerance *An investment term describing your ability to tolerate market downturns.*

Roth 401(k) *A newer form of 401(k) where tax is paid on the contributions, allowing all proceeds to be tax-free.*

search string *Text entry into a search engine to locate a topic on the web.*

seasonal assignment *Contracts issued, usually by facilities, to temporary healthcare workers for certain time periods during the year to cover increased patient census due to tourism or seasonal migration.*

shall *Contractual term used to indicate the person or party performing the work is responsible for the action stated.*

shared apartment *An apartment where two or more people are living.*

shift differential *Additional pay for working the 2nd or 3rd shift.*

show-stopper *Primary criteria you are not willing to compromise when selecting an agency.*

signature area *The area of a contract reserved for the signature of all parties.*

skills checklist *A self-evaluation form required by facilities and agencies describing your skill level for normal duties and procedures required by the assignment.*

sleep and rest requirement *An IRS acknowledgement of the need to be prepared for each day's work. Used to evaluate the tax-free status of some reimbursements.*

sole agency contract *A facility contracts with only one staffing agency to fill all of its needs.*

specialty agency *An agency that places only certain healthcare disciplines. Examples: dialysis or physical therapy.*

staffing agency *A business that provides facilities with healthcare workers on a temporary or permanent basis.*

standard clause *A legally worded contract clause appearing in all the agency's contracts describing a specific aspect of the agreement. Usually refers to general policy or procedures.*

state tax *The amount of yearly tax owed to one or more States.*

stipend *A negotiated amount paid to you, usually monthly, by an agency for use in acquiring your housing while on assignment.*

tax advantage program *Tax-free compensation offered to those that qualify under IRS rules for travel away from their permanent home.*

tax advisor *A person qualified to give tax advice and prepare your yearly tax returns.*

tax-free reimbursement *Those payments qualifying as tax-free under IRS criteria.*

tax home *The location the IRS considers your home for tax purposes.*

telephone interview *Usually your first contact with the facility. Used to clarify the working conditions and expectations prior to accepting an assignment.*

temporary assignment *An assignment lasting less than one year.*

temporary license *A short duration license issued by a State allowing you to begin work.*

tie-breaker *Secondary criteria used to evaluate and select agencies.*

time horizon *The time period until you begin to withdraw retirement funds.*

time sheet *Form submitted for pay indicating days and hours worked.*

TN status *Trade NAFTA status. Defined by the NAFTA treaty, streamlines the ability for residents of Canada and Mexico to gain entry to the U.S. for work purposes.*

toy hauler *A recreational vehicle with a large storage area used to transport equipment and smaller vehicles, such as ATV's, snow machines, etc.*

Traditional 401(k) *The original version of the 401(k). Contributions and proceeds are tax deferred until withdrawal.*

trailer *A living unit towed behind a vehicle.*

travel allowance *Payment for travel to and from an assignment. Usually tax-free if qualified.*

travel nurse *A healthcare worker willing to accept a temporary travel assignment. Usually requires a license to practice.*

traveler *Any healthcare worker willing to accept a temporary travel assignment.*

unfurnished apartment *An apartment for which you must provide all furnishings.*

vendor manager *A staffing agency acting on behalf of the facility to contract with other agencies to provide healthcare workers.*

visa screen *The process of evaluating a foreign applicant for entry into the U.S.*

W-4 form *Payroll withholding information form for Federal and State taxes.*

walk-through State *A State willing to issue a temporary license within a short period (usually one day) to those applying personally in their office.*

will *Contractual term used to indicate the person or party performing the work is not responsible for the action stated.*

Index